Releasing The Rotator Cuff

A complete guide to freedom of the shoulder

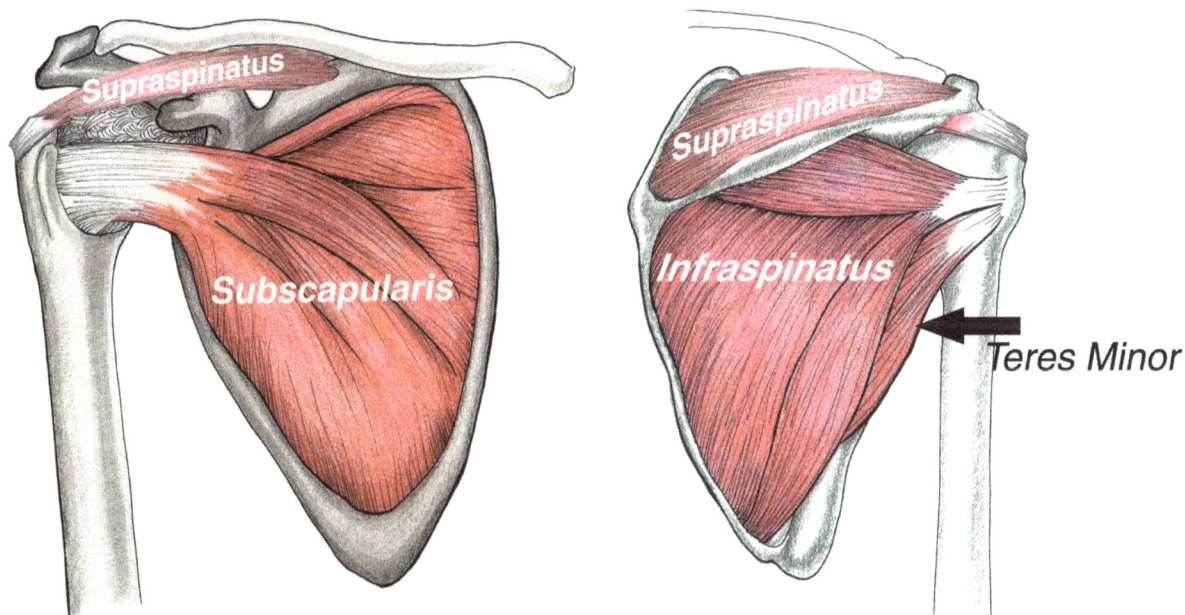

Supraspinatus

Subscapularis

Supraspinatus

Infraspinatus

Teres Minor

by
Peggy Lamb, MA, LMT, BCTMB

Drawings by Suzanne Dulany
Photographs by Grant Gurley, Jim Garon, and Kelly Page
Models: Nicki Dillon Gurley, Suzanne Dulany, Hope Malkan and Peggy Lamb

Additional copies of this book and other books and DVD's may be obtained from:
www.massagepublications.com

MASSAGE PUBLICATIONS
8400 Jamestown Dr #118
Austin, TX 78758
(512) 833-0179
info@massagepublications.com
Schools and distributors call or email for pricing.

**Thank you so much for purchasing
Releasing the Rotator Cuff!
There's a free thank you gift waiting for you at:
https://www.massagepublications.com**

Contents

Introduction

A number of years ago I injured my left rotator cuff during a yoga class. We were doing many sun salutations, which includes several poses that require the upper body to bear weight. My injury primarily involved tendonitis of the long head of the biceps, infraspinatus, and teres minor. Even though it was a minor injury it took over a year to heal and still bothers me at times today. The cause of my injury was not a trauma or blow to my shoulder but incorrect shoulder mechanics. This was a piece of humble pie to swallow since I teach body mechanics, dance and yoga classes! After analyzing my body mechanics I found that I was allowing my left shoulder to internally rotate during the poses that required me to bear weight on my arms and was also allowing my elbow to bend slightly instead of keeping it long, with the tip of the elbow rotated towards my midline. I'm sure that during one of the many movement-based classes I've taken someone had given a movement cue about this, (keeping the shoulder joint in external rotation when bearing weight on the arms), but it didn't penetrate my consciousness. I started paying more attention to this issue and, lo and behold, I tended to do just about everything, including massage, with my left shoulder slightly internally rotated. I went to fellow massage therapists for treatments, which helped, but I was disappointed that none of them educated me about shoulder mechanics. It was my chiropractor who suggested the excellent book, *The Seven Minute Rotator Cuff Solution* by Joseph Horrigan, D. C. and Jerry Robinson. I devoured this book and others and started my own rehabilitation of my rotator cuff, which included massage,strength training, stretching, chiropractic, and acupuncture. From my research and clinical experience I've discovered that 90 percent of all shoulder pain/rotator cuff dysfunction stem from incorrect shoulder mechanics.

Since then I've worked with hundreds of clients with rotator cuff injuries and have taught my techniques and protocols to thousands of massage therapists across the country. I believe we can give the best treatments when we have the "inside scoop" on a condition from our own healing journeys. It's always amazing how clients are attracted to us when we are ready to share our knowledge.

Often doctors will diagnose shoulder pain as bursitis or arthritis when the real problem is in the rotator cuff. Anti-inflammatory drugs are often prescribed which treats the symptoms but not the cause. Also, doctors may not make the patient aware that a simple change in sleeping position can be profoundly effective. My injury took a significant turn for the better when I changed from sleeping on my left affected side to sleeping on my right side. See the Client Education Section for more information on sleep position.

One client of mine was given an anti-inflammatory and sent to physical therapy where they had her doing strength training right away. She got worse and then her other shoulder began bothering her. It was too soon for her to do any strength training; restoration of a normal soft tissue environment through massage and stretching should have come before working with resistance. This is an all too familiar scenario.

There are first-rate physical therapy clinics and doctors, but, unfortunately there are some bad apples, too.

Another client with shoulder pain is wheel-chair bound and had a radical mastectomy many years ago. The combination of constantly sitting in a wheel-chair and the mastectomy deformed the connective tissue around her right chest to such a degree that the head of her right humerus has a sustained internal pull on it. She had terrible pain in her shoulder. The simple suggestion of sleeping with her shoulder *off* her pillow (she sleeps on her back) reduced her pain about 75 percent. Sleeping with her shoulder on the pillow subjected her poor shoulder to even more internal rotation. No wonder she was in pain! Yet her doctor only diagnosed it as arthritis and increased her pain medication.

A recent report[1] states that rotator cuff pathology is becoming more common in the fifth and sixth decades of life and almost 30% of visits to orthopedic clinics are for rotator cuff injuries. The report also states that more than 50% of individuals over 60 have at least a partial thickness rotator cuff tear and are among the most common of all orthopedic procedures. Yet many of these surgeries are unnecessary; non-invasive approaches such as the protocols in this book can be exceptionally effective.

I believe that client education (and cooperation) is the key to healing a rotator cuff injury. Quite often a massage therapist is the only health care practitioner who will take the time to look at the condition globally and provide the education necessary for a client's self care.

This book is a result of my research into rotator cuff injuries and teaching continuing education classes on the subject. It reflects my views* on the best way to treat them non-surgically. **This book is intended for mild to moderate injuries and improper use conditions. Anything more serious must be assessed by an osteopath, orthopedic specialist, or chiropractor**. It's my hope that this manual serves as a reference so you, the dedicated massage therapist, can pass the knowledge on to your clients. Please feel free to e-mail me with questions, comments, and feedback at info@massagepublications.com

[1] Kibler, W., Warme, B., Sciascia, A., Kuhn, J., & Wolf, B.(2009). Nonacute shoulder injuries. In W. Kibler (Ed.),Orthopedic knowledge update: Sports medicine (pp. 19–39) Rosemont, IL: American Academy of Orthopedic Surgeons.

*Students, clients, and colleagues have made valuable suggestions to this manual. All mistakes are mine alone.

Overview

The rotator cuff is a combination of four muscles (*supraspinatus, infraspinatus, teres minor, and subscapularis; commonly known as the "SITS" muscles*) that work to stabilize the head of the humerus during all shoulder movements (essentially most upper body movements). It keeps the humerus stable and centered in the shoulder joint. Think of them as guy wires pulling on a tent pole *(see graphic to your right)*:

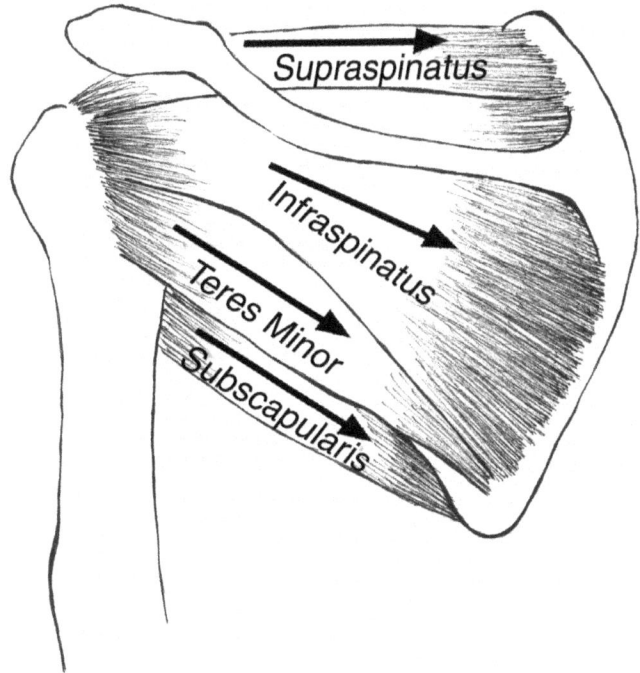

■The supraspinatus pulls the head of the humerus into the glenoid fossa from above.

■The infraspinatus pulls it in from the rear.

■The teres minor pulls it in from bottom/rear.

■The subscapularis pulls it in from the bottom/front.

Posterior view of rotator cuff muscles acting as guy wires holding the head of the humerus in.

The rotator cuff is the Commander-N-Chief of the shoulder – most shoulder conditions involves the rotator cuff in some way.

A healthy rotator cuff stabilizes the shoulder joint so we can do our activities of daily living without pain and swim, dance, play tennis, throw a ball, play golf etc.

In addition to serving this stabilizing function, the rotator cuff also counteracts the upward pull of the deltoid during abduction and flexion by pulling down and in on the head of the humerus. If it did not exert this downward/inward force, the head of the humerus would have an unpleasant collision with the acromion process of the scapula (the roof of the shoulder). It's quite a graceful duet if everything is working properly. We'll examine this in more detail in the lesson on shoulder mechanics.

Another way the rotator cuff works is as a decelerator. If you throw a ball or swing a tennis racket, first you externally rotate your shoulder as a wind up, then forcefully internally rotate as you throw or hit the ball. What keeps your arm from flying off your body? The ligaments of the shoulder and the rotator cuff, especially the infraspinatus and teres minor. These two small powerhouses are the only* external rotators of the

*Some authors include the posterior deltoid as an external rotator

shoulder joint. They have to work very hard to counterbalance the powerful internal rotators which outnumber them. *(There are five internal rotators of the shoulder joint: pectoralis major, anterior deltoid, subscapularis, latissimus dorsi and teres major.)*

In addition to the stabilizing and deceleration functions, the rotator cuff also performs movements:

Subscapularis: internal rotation
Infraspinatus and teres minor: external rotation of the humerus
Supraspinatus: abduction of the humerus

IN SUMMARY THE ROTATOR CUFF:

1. Stabilizes the head of the humerus during all shoulder joint movements.
2. Counteracts the upward pull of the deltoid during abduction and flexion of the humerus by exerting a downward pull on the head of the humerus.
3. Decelerates the arm when you throw something or swing a golf club, etc.
4. Provides movement: internal/external rotation and abduction of the humerus.

These are busy muscles that are constantly multitasking!

Of course the shoulder complex has quite a few ligaments supporting it also:

■ Acromioclavicular: acromion process to clavicle
■ Coracoacromial: coracoid process to acromion process
■ Coracoclavicular: coracoid process to clavicle
■ Coracohumeral: coracoid process to humerus
■ Glenohumeral: glenoid to humeral head

The rotator cuff is quite powerful in that it generates a force of 9.6 times the weight of the limb and generates maximum force at 60 degrees of abduction.

SIGNS OF AN INJURED ROTATOR CUFF:

Problems in the rotator cuff can manifest with a variety of symptoms. Most pain in the shoulder has something to do with the rotator cuff, either directly or indirectly.
Here's a partial list of the most common signs and symptoms:

■ Limited range of motion in the arm/shoulder. Limited external rotation and abduction is a typical pattern.

■ Pain in the upper arm, where the deltoid muscle is, especially when the arm is lifted away from the side in abduction. It may feel like the pain is deep in the shoulder joint. This pain is often from *trigger points* in the rotator cuff muscles and usually does not reflect pathology in the deltoid.

■ Pain at rest or during movement.

■   Pain during movements like those involved in getting dressed, brushing hair, reaching back to a night-stand, fastening a seat belt, putting on a coat and many more.

■   Weakness in the shoulder.

■   A clicking or popping sound when moving the arm.

■   A *painful arc* through part of the range of motion involved in abducting the humerus above the shoulder. This means you can move your arm without pain up to a certain point, then it hurts for a bit, then the pain goes away. This is called a painful arc.

ROTATOR CUFF INJURIES CAN INCLUDE ALL OR SOME OF THE FOLLOWING:

■   Tears in muscles and/or tendons.

■   Tendonitis or tendonosis (breakdown of collagen fibers) in tendons.

■   Trigger points in muscles.

■   Adaptive shortening of internal rotators.

■   Impingement of any of the structures that run through the space between the top of the humerus and bottom of the acromion (supraspinatus tendon, subacromial bursa and the long head of the biceps).

■   Formation of scar tissue (adhesions) that decrease the muscle's ability to contract and stretch. Scar tissue often binds together damaged and undamaged tissue, resulting in adhesions, causing pain, re-injury, and restricted range of movement. Scar tissue primarily forms in ligaments, muscles, tendons, fascia, and joint capsules.

■   Injury such as a fall onto the shoulder.

■   Bicipital tendonitis (inflammation of the long head of the biceps) which sometimes accompanies rotator cuff injuries.

Usually, the real problem is ***dysfunctional shoulder mechanics***. Ninety percent of all rotator cuff injuries arise from:

- Strength imbalance between internal and external rotators.

- Weak and overstretched external rotators.

- Adaptively shortened internal rotators.

- Weak scapulae stabilizers (serratus anterior, rhomboids, lower and middle traps etc). If the scapula is not correctly positioned the scapulohumeral muscles will not be able to maintain their optimal length-tension relationships.

PEOPLE AT RISK:

Carpenters, athletes; people with internally rotated shoulders, collapsed chest and forward neck posture; golfers; massage therapists (yes, that means you!); weight lifters; swimmers; occupations requiring heavy lifting; people who carry heavy bags (laptops, backpacks, etc.); and anyone who does repetitive motions at the joint, especially overhead motions.

Unless you are a sports massage therapist or have a practice that specializes in athletes, the majority of rotator cuff injuries you'll see will be in clients who don't play professional baseball, but have injured their rotator cuff because of improper shoulder mechanics, especially those clients over the age of 45 when the wear and tear starts showing up.

A Lesson In Shoulder Mechanics

The shoulder girdle and shoulder joint:
The shoulder girdle is the scapulae and clavicles. The shoulder or glenohumeral joint is where the head of the humerus fits into the glenoid fossa created by the shoulder girdle. Although these are separate joints, they work together most of the time.

Movements of the shoulder girdle (scapulae and clavicles): elevation, depression, retraction, protraction, upward and downward rotation.

Movements of the shoulder joint: abduction, adduction, lateral (external) rotation, medial (internal) rotation, flexion, extension, circumduction.

BONES OF THE SHOULDER GIRDLE AND JOINT

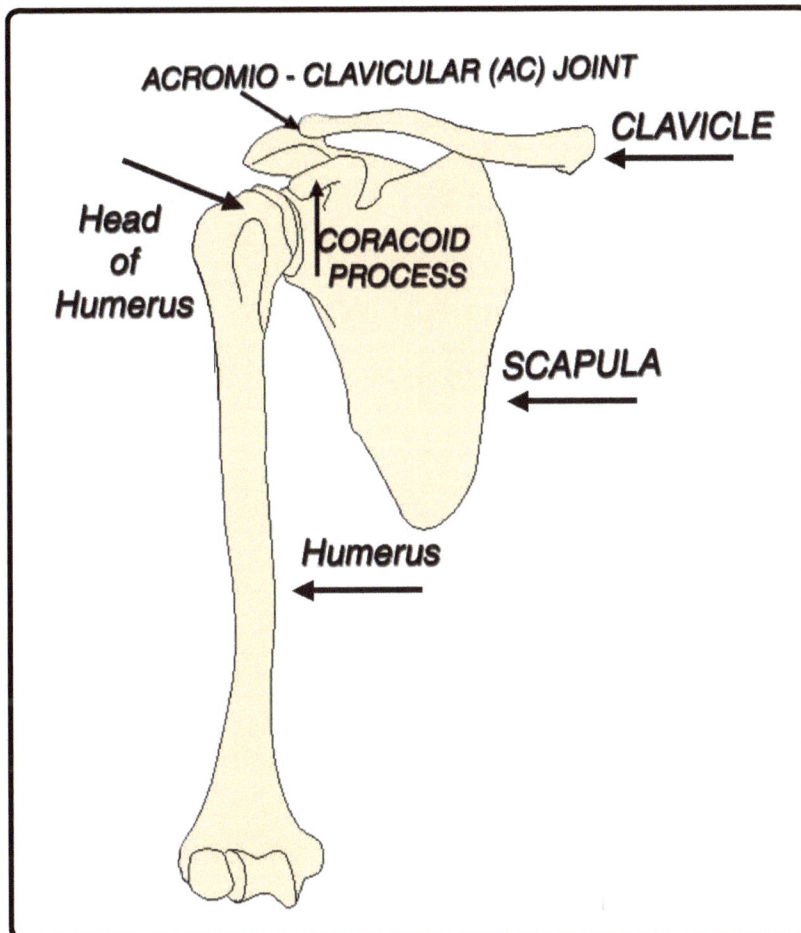

ANTERIOR VIEW

SCAPULOHUMERAL RHYTHM:

The shoulder girdle and shoulder joint dance a lovely duet called the scapulohumeral rhythm. In order for the humerus to move past 90 degrees of abduction and 45 to 60 degrees of flexion, the scapula must move in order to accommodate the humerus. Upward and downward rotation of the scapula happens when the humerus is abducted higher than 90 degrees or flexed higher than 60 degrees. We'll use abduction as our model.

Figure A shows the humerus abducted to 30 degrees and the scapula in neutral. As the humerus rises toward 90 degrees, the head of the humerus approaches the acromion process. In order to abduct the humerus higher than 90 degrees, the scapula must get out of the way, or else the head of the humerus would collide with the acromion process.

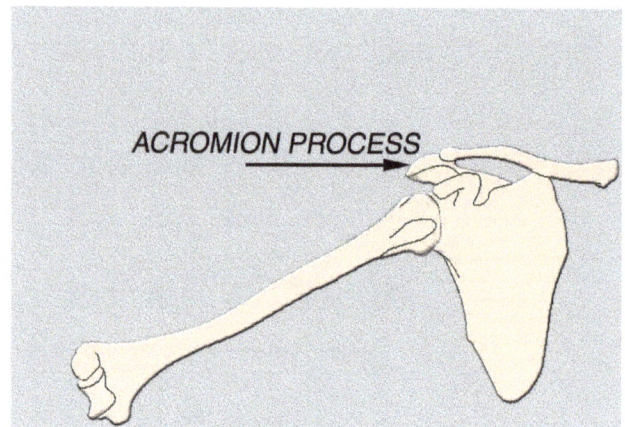

Figure A

Figure B shows the scapula upwardly rotated, leaving a clear pathway for the head of the humerus. The dark gray scapula in **Figure B** shows the scapula in neutral. Upward rotation refers to the acromion process, clavicle, and glenoid fossa rotating upward. Feel it on yourself by placing your fingers in the middle of your clavicle and walking your fingers laterally till it meets with the acromion process.

Now abduct your arm above 90 degrees and you will feel the acromion process and clavicle upwardly rotating.

The trapezius and serratus anterior are the prime movers for upward rotation of the scapula. Since these two muscles tend to be locked short (held in a concentric contraction), they are likely candidates for impeding healthy rotator cuff function. If the scapula cannot upwardly rotate in time because of dysfunction in these two muscles, micro-tearing of tissue, especially the supraspinatus, occurs.

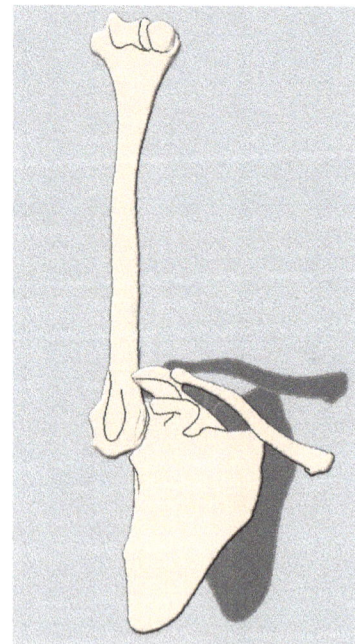

Figure B

It is in the range of movement from 60° to 180° that many folks with problematic rotator cuffs have difficulty. This is usually caused by impingement of the supraspinatus tendon, the long head of the biceps or the subacromial bursa, perhaps from too many years of abducting the humerus while it's internally rotated.

Now let's consider that nasty and pervasive habit of letting the shoulders roll forward into internal rotation. Study **Figure C** below and notice the position of the greater tubercle. Find it on yourself by first locating the lesser tubercle which is the first bump you'll find on your anterior shoulder. You will feel a di[...] [...] bercle. You're in the groove now - the bicipital groove [...] of the biceps. Do a little cross fiber friction on that te[...] groove and you'll feel another, larger bump. You're o[...] supraspinatus tendon which is located on the upper [...] use cross fiber friction on it. Is yours talking to you?

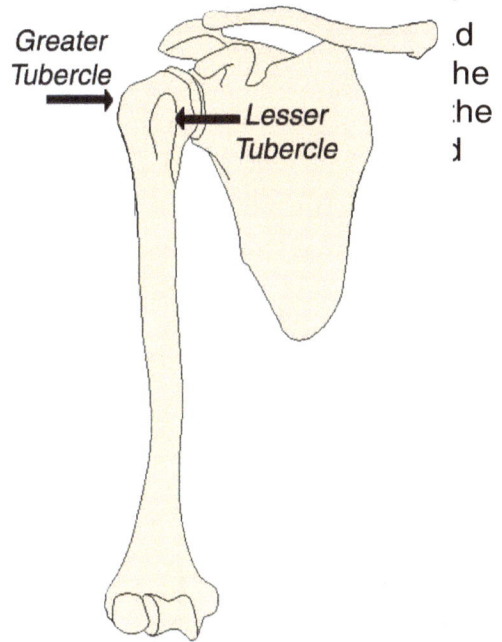

Figure C
(Anterior View)

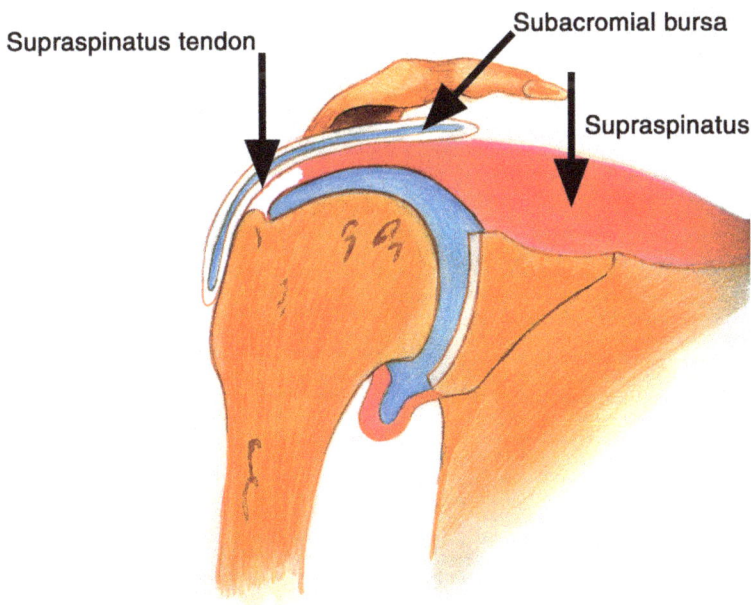

Figure D
(Anterior View)

Figure D, left, shows the humerus in a neutral position. Notice that the clavicle has been removed to better show the structures of the supraspinatus muscle and tendon, and the subacromial bursa.

When the humerus is internally rotated, the greater tubercle rolls forward, taking that supraspinatus tendon and the tendons of the infraspinatus and teres minor along for the ride. Since the supraspinatus attaches to the top of the greater tubercle, it will collide with the acromion process if the humerus is abducted in the internally rotated position as shown in *Figure E*.

Try it out on yourself and you'll feel the restriction of the greater tubercle colliding with the acromion process. Just imagine how many times people do this on any given day! You can see why this muscle/tendon unit is so frequently torn and/or impinged as shown in *Figure F* on the next page.

Surgical repair may be necessary to restore function. In fact, this superior aspect of the shoulder joint is called the impingement area. The subacromial bursa lies above the supraspinatus and underneath the acromion process and, of course, it too suffers from irritation and inflammation when impinged.

The optimum alignment for the great tubercle to glide under the acromium during abduction is 30-45 degrees forward of the frontal plane (scaption).

The moral of this story: **Always abduct with the thumb up!**

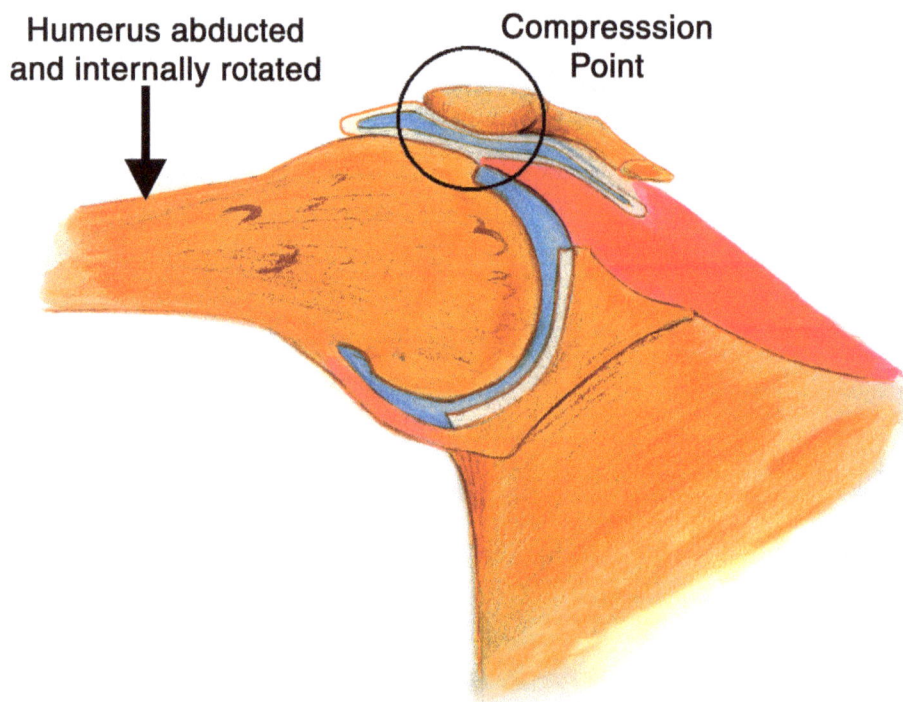

Humerus abducted
and internally rotated

Compresssion
Point

Figure E
(Anterior View)

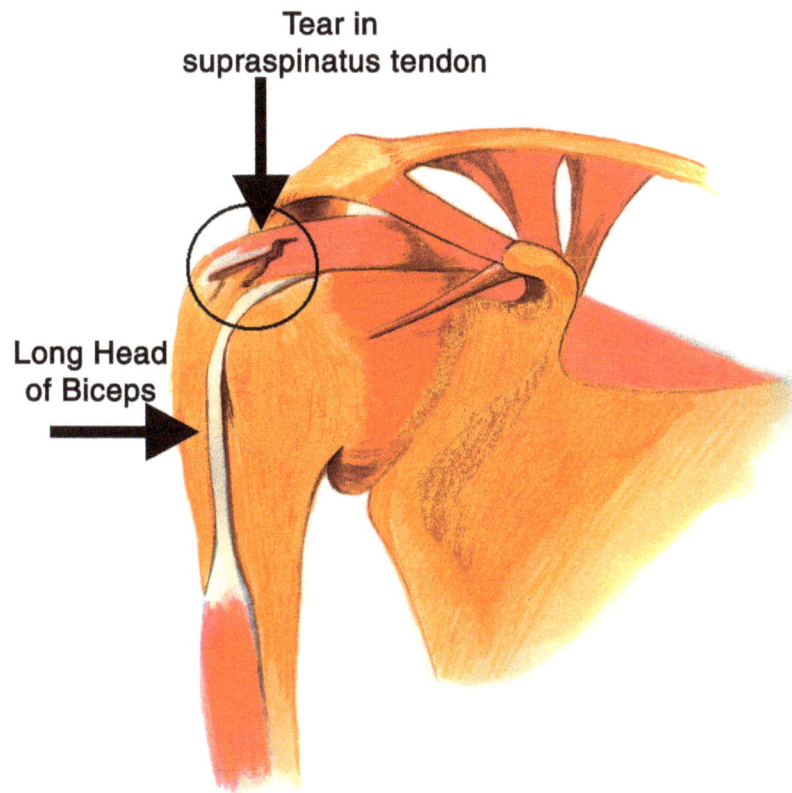

Figure F
(Anterior View)

Let's turn our attention to the long head of the biceps *(the short head of the biceps has been cut out of **Figure F**)*. Habitual internal rotation will cause that tendon to rub against either the lesser or greater tubercles causing micro-tearing, impingement, and inflammation.

Internal rotation is our friend! It allows us to do many movements. But it is not a friendly position to call "home." Home position for bones should be in neutral. In neutral, our wonderful bones can be the weight supporting structures they were designed for and transfer weight through the center of the joints. With our bones centered in their proper homes, our muscles can cease to be weight supporting structures, giving them the freedom to move our bones and allowing us to move with greater ease and vitality and to express ourselves through our bodies.

MORE ABOUT IMPINGEMENT SYNDROME:

HAWKINS-KENNEDY IMPINGEMENT SIGN: If you suspect impingement syndrome, you can test for it easily. Flex the client's shoulder to 90 degrees and from that position, internally rotate and horizontally adduct, (bring the arm across the chest), the humerus as far as it will go. This brings the greater tuberosity of the humerus up under the cora-coacromial arch and it will press on the soft tissue structures under the arch (supraspinatus tendon, long head of biceps and subacromial bursa.) If impingement syndrome is present, this test will reproduce the pain/discomfort. If you have a client that is not responding to treatment, they may have a Type II or Type III acromion process. In Type II, the acromion process is curved and dips downward; Type III acromion processes are beaked. Both types obstruct the outlet for the supraspinatus tendon. This can easily be seen with an X-Ray. Surgery may be the best option, especially for Type III's.

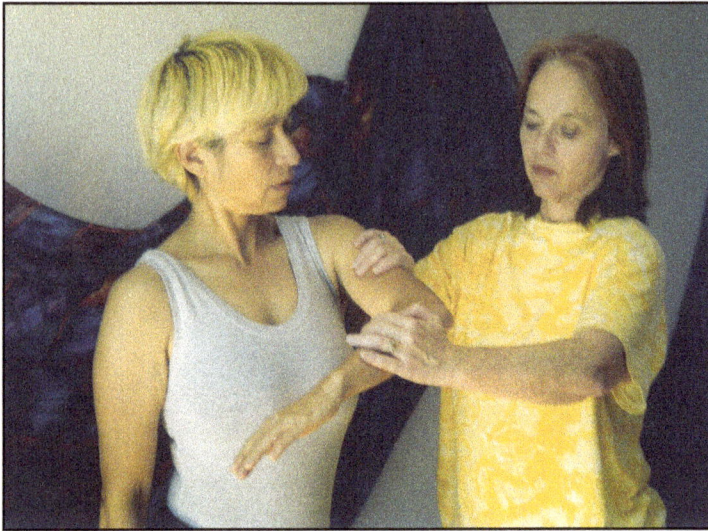

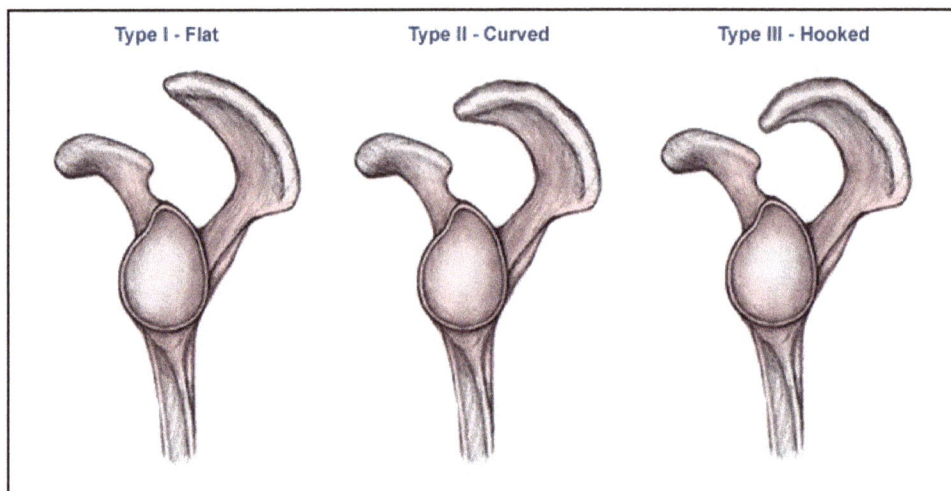

| Type I - Flat | Type II - Curved | Type III - Hooked |

My personal experience with impingement syndrome is that it responds well to good, precise deep tissue work on all the muscles presented in this book, especially serratus anterior and upper trapezius, along with ultra sound, acupuncture, ice, stretching and the Pendulum Exercise (see Client Education Section). Mine came on suddenly after a camping trip and it took a good year to resolve. My range of motion was always good, even in the worst of it. Abduction and horizontal adduction were the most painful movements for me.

ASSESSMENT TESTS

The following assessment tests are useful in pointing you in the right direction. For example, if I find that the scapula is not gliding smoothly on the thorax when I do the Scapula Glide/Scapulohumeral Rhythm Test, I will spend more time in my first session on serratus anterior, subscapularis, trapezius and pectoralis minor - muscles that can cause glueing and locking of the scapula on the thorax.

The shoulder is an intricate area and these tests are by no means definitive. Your client may need further testing by a physical or occupational therapist. When in doubt, refer out!

Muscle Testing:

Purpose: to evaluate the available range of motion of the shoulder complex and the strength of the rotator cuff muscles.

Protocol: Before beginning your treatments, have your client move her shoulder through her available range of motion. This gives you a baseline reading for comparison in subsequent sessions.

You can then test each muscle by having your client do its movement against resistance that you provide. Pain and/or weakness can indicate pathology in the muscle. The client is standing in each of the following tests.

Supraspinatus: have your client abduct the arm to 90 degrees (or less if 90 degrees is painful), then apply a moderate downward pressure on the humerus while the client tries to maintain the abduction.

Infraspinatus/Teres Minor: to test for external rotation, the humerus should be in neutral (at the client's side) with the elbow bent to 90 degrees. Have her externally rotate the humerus while you provide resistance to the back of the forearm.

Subscapularis: to test for internal rotation, have your client place her hand against the upper abdomen, just under the xyphoid process. Ask her to press as hard as she can into the abdomen by internally rotating the shoulder. The test is positive if your client flexes the wrist and adducts and extends the shoulder, instead of internally rotating the shoulder.

Keep in mind that although a muscle may test as strong, there still may be and often are trigger points and adhesions in the tissue.

There are many good books on muscle testing that offer more in-depth information and techniques.

Scapula Glide/Scapulohumeral Rhythm Test:

Purpose: to evaluate how easily the scapula glides on the thorax and determine the synchrony of the scapulohumeral rhythm. To check for winged scapula.

Protocol: to get a baseline reading, place your hand on the scapula of the unaffected shoulder. Ask your client to abduct her arm above her shoulder. You hand should swivel as the scapula upwardly rotates. Feel for the smooth gliding of the scapula on the thorax. Notice *how* your client abducts her arm. Is her shoulder joint internally rotated? If so, you've just learned a perpetuating factor. Use this assessment as a teaching tool about healthy shoulder mechanics. **Always abduct with the thumb up!**

Repeat this test on the affected side. Again, notice *how* your client abducts her arm. If the scapula is not gliding or moving easily, this can indicate a problem in the scapulohumeral rhythm. Possible causes are trigger points and adhesions in the upward rotators of the scapula (serratus anterior and trapezius) or trigger points and adhesions in the subscapularis which causes the scapula to become glued or locked on the thorax.

Repeat this test on the both sides simultaneously to compare and confirm your findings.

A winged or protruding scapula will most likely disrupt the scapulohumeral rhythm. A winged scapula is associated with damage or a contusion to the long thoracic nerve of the shoulder and / or weakness in the serratus anterior muscle. If the long thoracic nerve is damaged or bruised it can cause paralysis of the serratus anterior muscle and winging of the scapula. If the condition does not respond to your treatment please refer to a physical or occupational therapist.

GUIDELINES FOR MANUAL THERAPISTS:

1. I suggest first releasing the muscles that are locked-short* (subscapularis, supraspinatus, pectoralis major etc.). This allows the bones to find their "home base" and takes some of the load off the muscles that are locked long. Massage all affected muscles and tendons using direct compression, effleurage, friction, etc.

2. Release trigger points through deep stroking and/or direct compression on the specific point. The subject of trigger points is a big one and beyond the scope of this book. I recommend Drs. Travell and Simons masterful two volume set, *Myofascial Pain and Dysfunction - The Trigger Point Manual*, or Clair Davies excellent *The Trigger Point Therapy Workbook*.

3. Retire Attila the Thumb and go *"muscle swimming"* using active movement. With active movement we utilize muscle physiology to slowly swim through the muscles' barriers and layers. For example, have your client internally and externally rotate her shoulder joint while you press on a trigger point in subscapularis. You'll be amazed how the muscle organically releases. It's a win-win situation. The active movement lessens the pain and discomfort for your client and you save your hands. (See Principles of Muscle Swimming section for more detailed instructions.)

4. Muscles release best when worked in shortened, neutral and stretched states.

5. Work and release the muscles from supine, side-lying and prone positions (not necessarily in that order). This comprehensive approach is extremely effective. I usually start people supine and work all the muscles from supine, then do my side-lying work and finally my prone work. However, each client and situation is different. Adapt my techniques and protocols to meet you and your client's needs.

6. Stretch all internal rotators (pectoralis major, anterior deltoid, subscapularis, latissimus dorsi, and teres major.)

7. Educate client about proper shoulder mechanics; modify sleeping position (many people re-injure their rotator cuff from improper sleeping positions. See Client Education Section), modify or eliminate certain exercises such as bench-presses. A more complete guide to the modification of exercises and which ones to avoid can be found in the excellent book, *The Seven Minute Rotator Cuff Solution* by Joseph Horrigan, D. C. and Jerry Robinson.

When a muscle is locked-short, it is being held in a concentric or shortened state. Locked-long means that the muscle is being held in an eccentric or stretched state.

8. In addition to releasing the rotator cuff muscles and all internal rotators, it is imperative to also address the serratus anterior, pectoralis minor, biceps and trapezius muscles.

9. Ask your client, *"what is the one movement or activity that you have the most trouble with or that you'd like to be able to do pain-free?"* This question usually yields a gold mine of information and clients feel cared about. One client of mine answered this question with *"I just want to be able to hold my IPhone!"*

10. Apply cold or moist heat packs to affected muscles (either before or after working them, or both).

11. Hydration: advise your clients to drink plenty of water as poorly hydrated tissue impedes healing.

12. I've put together a fabulous *"From Ouch to Aaah!" Shoulder Pain Self-Care* book which allows your clients to "take you home" with them and extend the benefits of your healing touch while they are at home. For more information go to the link below:

https://www.massagepublications.com/from-ouch-to-aaah/

TREATMENT OBJECTIVES:

1. Reduction of pain and inflammation.
2. Restoration of a normal soft tissue environment.
3. Restoration of normal range of motion.

■ Allow at least an hour and a half to two hours for the first session.

■ Subsequent sessions will vary in length depending on your clients condition.

■ Work according to your client's pressure tolerance releasing the superficial layers of the tissue first.

■ If your client shows no improvement after four sessions, refer to an osteopath, family doctor, orthopedic specialist, or chiropractor.

■ The number of treatments depends on the severity* of the condition and how long the condition has been present. I suggest starting with one or two times per week for four weeks and reassessing after that. Regularity of treatment is essential for improvement.

■ If your work worsens the condition (not just post-massage soreness) refer your client to a doctor.

Some conditions require more aggressive interventions than massage therapists can provide. Your client may have torn ligaments, damage to the joint capsule, subacromial bursitis, arthritis, etc. If someone presents with extreme pain, muscle wasting, or other obvious signs of nerve or disc damage, refer them immediately to a doctor. When in doubt, refer out!

CONTRAINDICATIONS

1. Hypermobile shoulders
2. Shoulder replacements
2. Breast cancer/ lymphedema: this is a contraindication specific to subscapularis work. Align yourself with an Occupational Therapist with an expertise in working with breast cancer.
3. Bursitis: this is a contraindication specific to supraspinatus work. Avoid the lateral section of the muscle/tendon unit.

Frozen Shoulder:
Frozen shoulder or adhesive capsulitis is when the joint capsule adheres to the humeral head. This condition can be secondary to another shoulder injury, including rotator cuff dysfunction, but can also occur without any discernible trauma or trigger. I believe thoughtful, careful massage of the muscles presented in this manual can be an effective treatment for frozen shoulder. Be conservative about passive and active stretching, as it may exacerbate the symptoms. For a more detailed description of this condition see Ruth Werner's excellent article, *Adhesive Capsulitis: Freezing, Frozen, Thawing Shoulders*, in the May 2003 issue of *Massage Today*.

http://www.massagetoday.com/mpacms/mt/article.php?id=10708

PRINCIPLES OF MUSCLE SWIMMING

As manual therapists we all face the question, "How can I best facilitate tissue release and allow the muscle to return to its happy, healthy resting state while maintaining my own ecology of movement?" I stumbled across an answer to that dilemma about twelve years ago and have been refining my approach ever since in both my private practice and seminars. Simply put, Muscle Swimming uses physiology to facilitate release of myofascial structures allowing the therapist to work smarter and the client to have co-ownership of the session. The following are the core components of Muscle Swimming:

1. Warm the tissue with Swedish strokes before deep tissue work.

2. **Pin and Rock:** our first encounter with a stressed myofascial unit should be gentle and non-threatening. Passively shorten the muscle and gently pin it with multiple fingers for a broad, dispersed pressure. Then add a slow rhythmic rocking of the joint. Rocking stimulates a parasympathetic response. After all, we are rocked for nine months. In fact, the first nerves to myelinate in the human fetus are the vestibular nerves which sense movement. Our first consciousness is that we are a moving beings. Be patient – wait for the tissue to soften and yield before moving to the Pin and Move protocol. Come back to this Pin and Rock maneuver whenever you sense guarding in your client.

3. **Pin and Move:** when you meet an area of dense fascia, trigger points, tender points or just plain snarly tissue, integrate active movement. Active movement "takes it to the brain", involving the central nervous system, creating longer lasting results. Fascial layers and actin and myosin myofibrils glide across each other as the muscle goes through its shortened, neutral and stretched states.
   A. Place the muscle in a shortened state.
   B. Pin the area at first barrier. If it's a trigger point or tender point, use one finger, or appropriate tool for specificity and work from an oblique angle of 45 degrees.
   C. Have your client do a movement. Start with the main action the muscle performs, i.e. flexion, abduction, extension etc. Movement should be done at a slow to medium tempo.
   D. Client repeats the movement 4-5 times.
   E. Ask your client if the area or point is better, worse or the same. If your client says that the area is better, your nest question is, "how much better?" If your client reports at least a 50% change for the better, then move to another area and repeat the above steps.
   F. If your client reports no change you have three options:
     1. Add resistance to the current movement pattern. This loads the muscle and recruits more fibers, allowing you to swim through the tissue.

10 - 20% of resistance is usually all that is needed. For example, your client is performing internal and external rotations of the shoulder joint while you pin a stubborn trigger point in the subscapularis. To add resistance, having your client press into your hand or arm. I keep one and three pound weights under my table and put one in my client's hand if I need to recruit more muscle fibers with active-resisted movement. If you don't have weights, a can of soup or a small bottle of water will do!

       2. Try another movement pattern. Adding resistance to the new pattern is always an option.
       3. Ask your client for input. She may feel an itch to move the joint in a certain way.

       G. If your client reports that the point or area is worse that's not necessarily a negative outcome. It's possible that through the portal of Active Movement, you've swum to a trigger point or congested area at a deeper layer of tissue.
The same three options apply to this situation as well:

       1. Add resistance to the current movement pattern.
       2. Try another movement pattern. Adding resistance to the new pattern is always an option.
       3. Ask your client for input. She may feel an itch to move the joint in a certain way.

4. Work the muscle(s) from as many different positions as possible — supine, side-lying, prone, and even weight-bearing. Perhaps your client is a golfer suffering with stubborn trigger points in the infraspinatus. Have him go through a golf swing while you work the tissue. Think outside the box and get the client moving!

5. When you find an exquisitely tender spot or trigger point, work to release the tissue around it before concentrating on the tender point.

6. Give your client a break! Working on these muscles, especially the iliopsoas, can be quite stressful. Incorporate what I call the "sweet stuff" during your deep tissue work, i.e., energy work, a short foot massage, some relaxing effleurage, etc.

7. Breath connects us all! Breathe deeply while working and encourage your client to do the same.

8. Combine working two muscles at the same time. Since all muscles work interdependently this is an especially effective release technique.

9. Practice patience, non-judgment, curiosity, and compassion.

10. If it hurts you, don't do it! Adapt the technique to suit your body.

Rotator Cuff Muscles

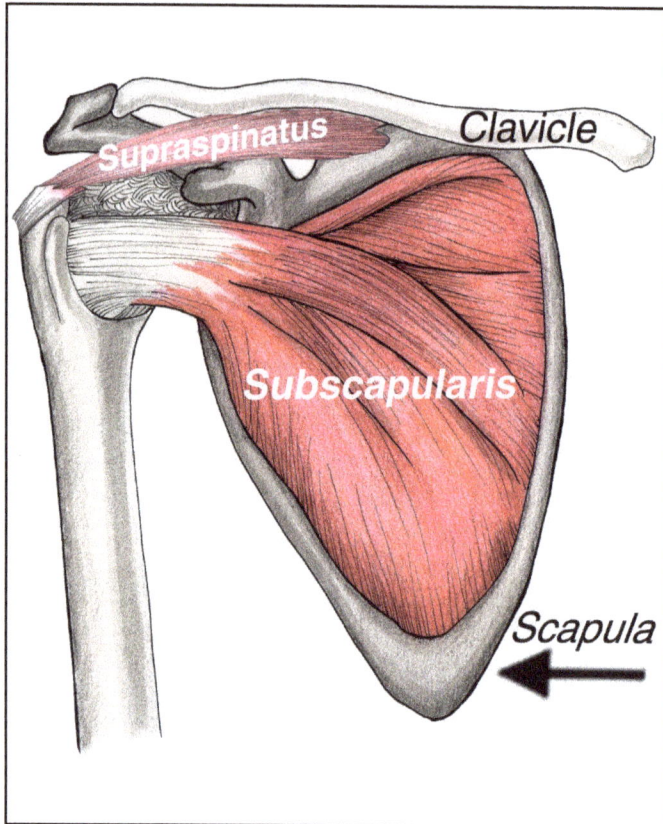

Supraspinatus

Clavicle

Subscapularis

Scapula

Anterior View

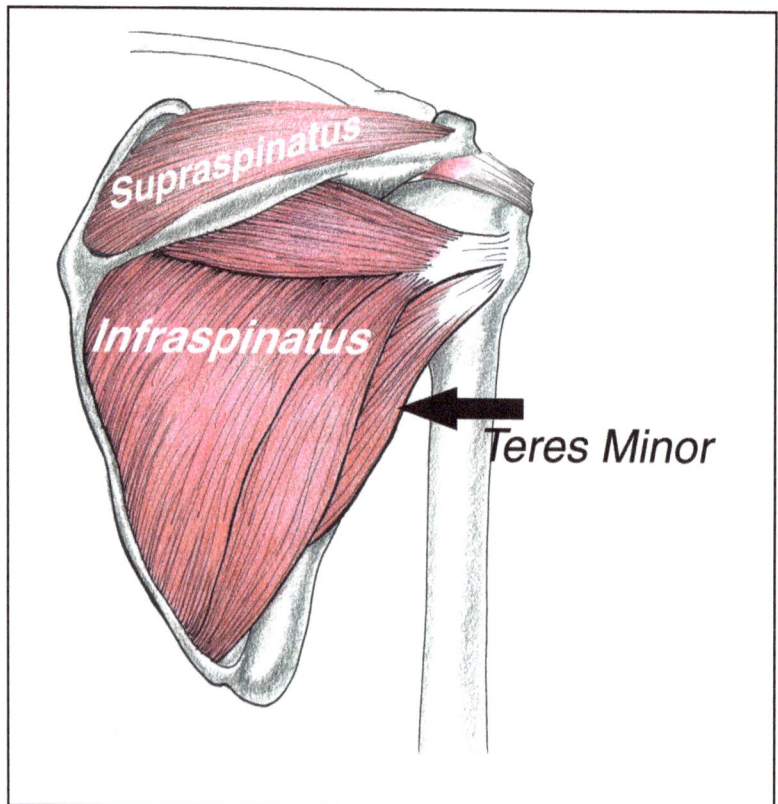

Supraspinatus

Infraspinatus

Teres Minor

Posterior View

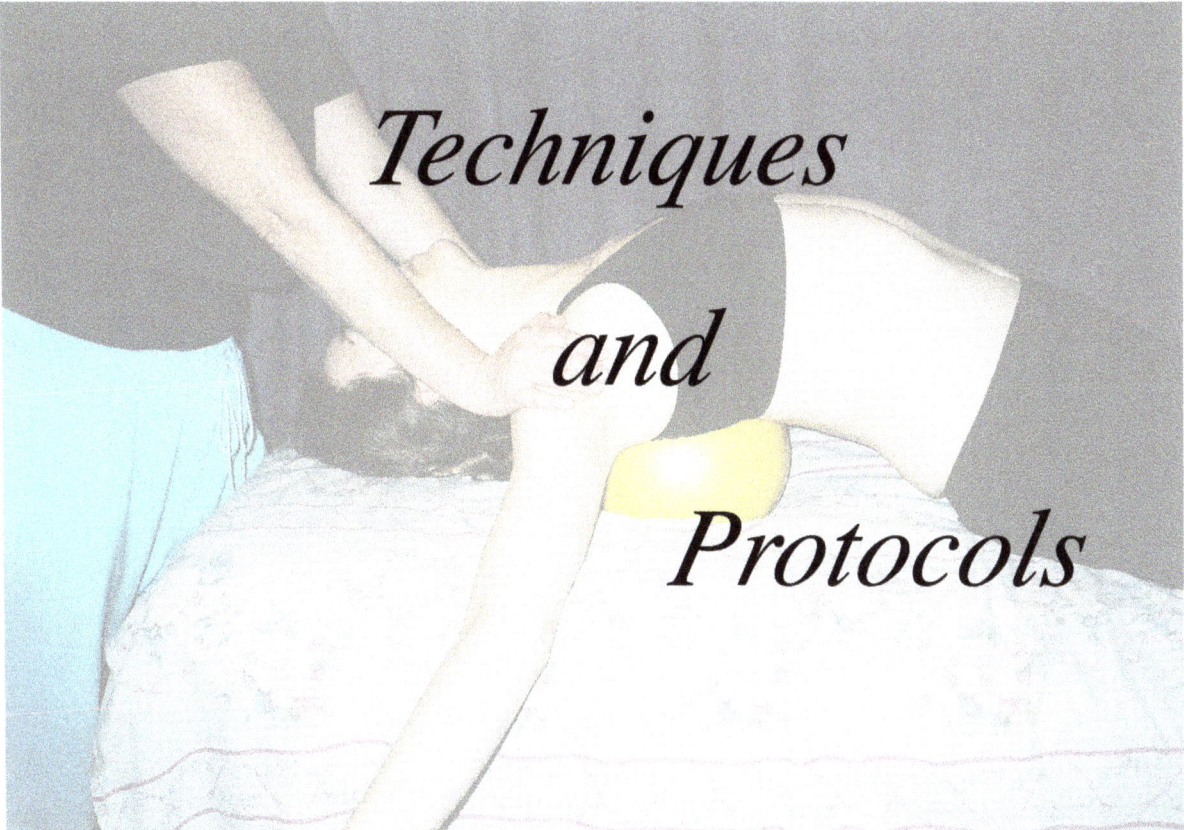

Techniques
and
Protocols

The following pages present techniques and protocols for releasing the rotator cuff and surrounding musculature. The **X's** on the drawings represent the most common sites of trigger points, although I have found trigger points can be anywhere. These techniques and protocols are *"a way"* not *"the way"* and are there to serve as guidelines or trail markers. The muscles do not have to be worked in the order presented. It's practical to do all your supine or prone work at the same time. Do stretch the muscle after you work it. This is when the muscle is most responsive. Each client is unique and presents us with creative challenges in the use of our skills, intuition and knowledge. Neck problems contribute to shoulder problems, therefore it is wise to release the neck before beginning the shoulder work. Expand and enlarge upon the following techniques and protocols with your knowledge and creativity. Know the actions and attachments of the muscle you are working. A strong foundational knowledge of anatomy is indispensable for intelligent, intuitive bodywork. Below are a few images or sayings I think about when doing bodywork:

- Dance with the muscles!

- Combine working two muscles at the same time. Since all muscles work interdependently, especially the rotator cuff, this is an especially effective release technique.

- Work the muscle in a shortened state, a neutral state, and a stretched state.

- Tire the muscle, don't tear it!

- How can I do this more softly? (Not necessarily less pressure)

- Allow your fingers to "swim" gently and deeply through the tissue layers.

- Experiment with traction and compression while working the muscles.

- Breath connects us all! Breathe deeply while working and encourage your client to do the same.

- Practice patience, non-judgment, curiosity, and compassion.

- If it hurts you, don't do it! Adapt the technique to suit your body.

- Feel before acting and follow the cues of the client.

- The healer in you contacts the healer in your client.

- Save your hands! Use tools. Small hot stones are wonderful, especially for the small supraspinatus.

SUBSCAPULARIS MUSCLE

Actions: internal rotation of the humerus at the shoulder joint and stabilization of the head of humerus in the glenoid fossa. Also assists in adduction of the humerus.
Attachments: medial border of the anterior surface of the scapula and the lesser tubercle of the humerus.

The subscapularis is a thick muscle with a broad tendon which covers the anterior scapula and reinforces the shoulder joint. It functions to stabilize, internally rotate, depress and adduct the humeral head in the glenoid fossa. Attachments are the medial border of the anterior surface of the scapula and the lesser tubercle of the humerus.

This sturdy muscle provides 50% of the strength of the rotator cuff. Subscap plays a vital role in joint centration, depressing the humeral head, along with the other rotator cuff muscles, during abduction of the shoulder joint, counteracting the powerful force of the deltoid. Weakness, or as I like to think of it, disruption of its ability to function at full capacity, can lead to anterior glide syndrome, as the larger internal rotators drive the humeral head anterior, which often leads to impingement syndrome. Another important function of subscap is its eccentric activity, protecting the shoulder joint during external rotation.

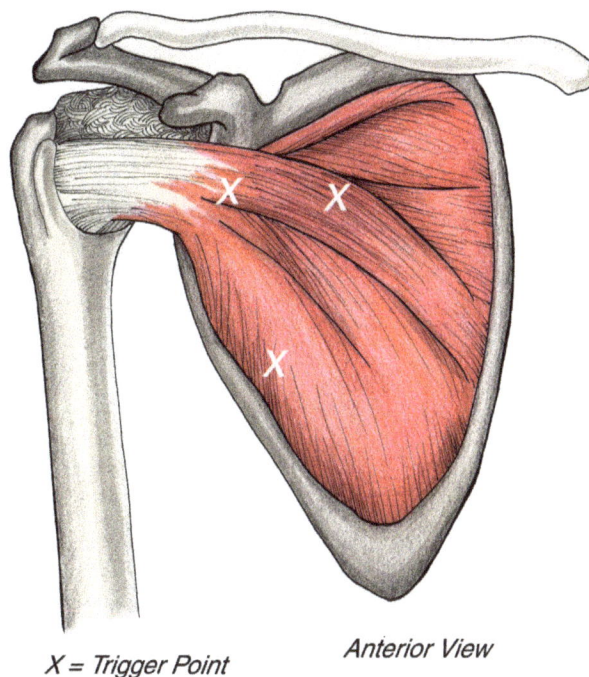

X = Trigger Point

Anterior View

The scapula rests on the serratus anterior and subscap, which move across one another as the scapula moves so working on these muscles assists the scapula to glide on the thorax.

The shoulder joint follows the scapula. Increasing scapula stability and mobility leads to increased glenohumeral joint function. Skilled comprehensive work on subscap is essential for recovery from rotator injuries.

Trigger points the refer across the shoulder blade, down the arm, and around the wrist.

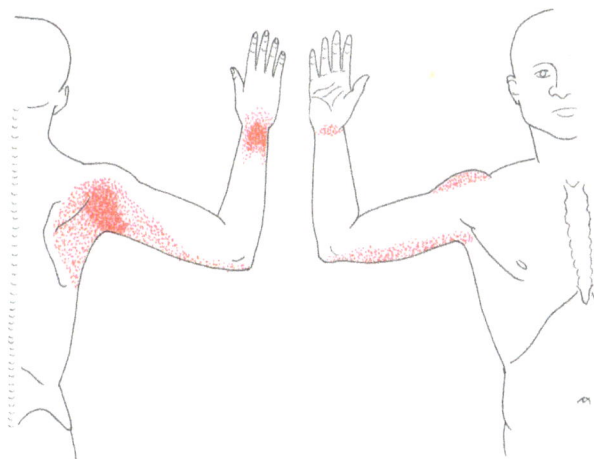

PALPATION

In my workshops I've discovered that approximately 80% of therapists thought they were on subscap, but were on latissimus dorsi/teres major. It's an easy mistake to make and easily correctable. The reason for this common error is that therapists attempt to enter subscap too far inferiorly. If you do that the ribs will block you and you will mistake the fat lat for subscap.

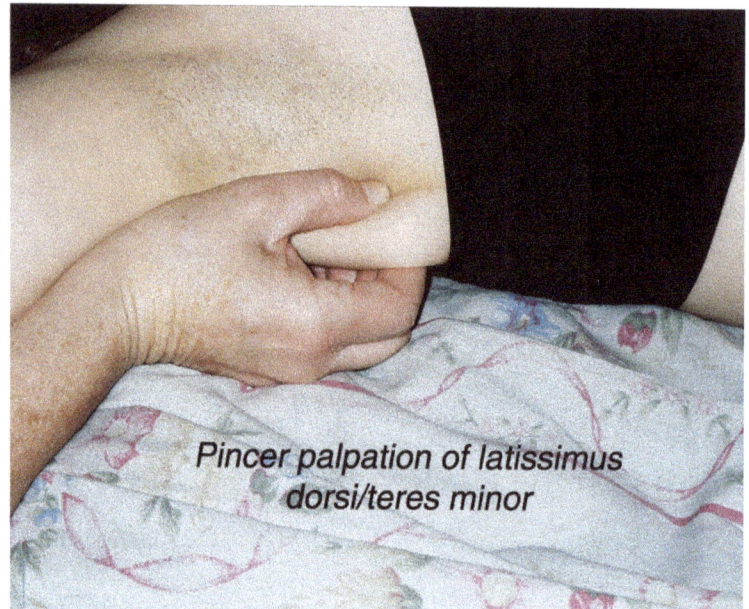

Pincer palpation of latissimus dorsi/teres minor

The best place to enter subscap territory is the central portion of the muscle. Bear with me while I use this analogy. I live in beautiful Austin, which is in central Texas. Dallas is north and San Antonio is south. If I try to enter subscap in the San Antonio area, I'll most likely mistake latissimus dorsi for subscap. If I enter in the Dallas area, I'll probably hit the tendon, which is fine if that's where I want to start. I prefer to enter through Austin, which puts me in the less sensitive central belly and I can glide superior or inferior from there. (That's assuming the client's scapula is not super-glued to the thorax, which it often is. More about that later.)

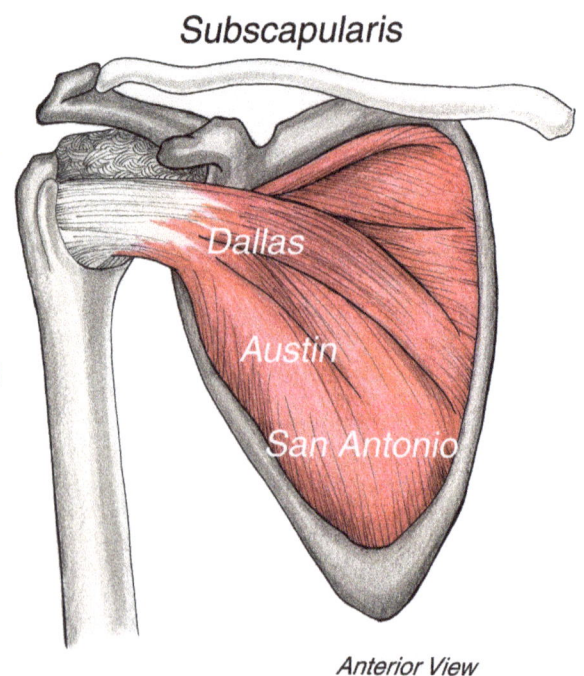

Subscapularis

Dallas

Austin

San Antonio

Anterior View

24

Staying with this analogy, substitute your cities for mine. Begin your entry into subscap from your city. Dive under pec major with your fingers to get your medial placement first and only then gently press your finger tips toward the scapula. The medial placement is crucial, pressing posteriorly too soon causes the fingers to slide laterally and you'll wind up on lat.

Verify your location by sliding your fingers laterally to feel the lateral border of the scapula. If you are lateral to the lateral border of the scapula, you are on latissimus/teres major, not subscap. Your mantra is:
To accurately palpate subscap your fingers must be medial to the lateral border of the scapula!

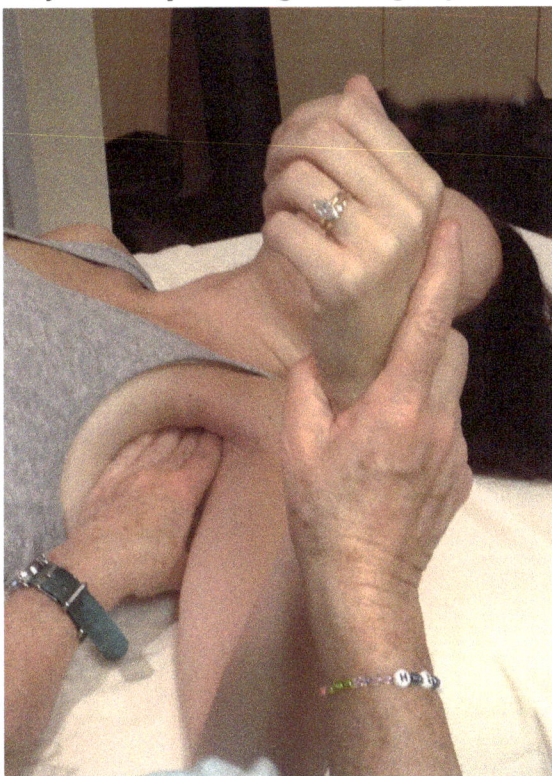

STRATEGIES FOR WORKING WITH SUBSCAP

It's all about the principles! "As to methods there may be a million and then some, but principles are few. The man who grasps principles can successfully select his own methods. The man who tries methods, ignoring principles is sure to have trouble." (Harrington Emerson)

I think of subscap as the psoas of the shoulder because of its sensitivity, the feeling of vulnerability it evokes in the client and its propensity to stimulate a sympathetic nervous response. Positional release and rocking are two excellent strategies to make subscap work more palatable for the client.

Work this muscle in all three positions: supine, side-lying and prone. Each position offers its own advantage. I think it's best to begin work on subscap in the supine position for several reasons. The resting length of the muscle can be assessed by noting if the client's wrist contacts the table when the humerus is externally rotated and abducted with the elbow bent to 90 degrees (humerus is in "L" shape). If it doesn't, that's a sure sign of a shortened subscapularis. Supine is a good position to release several of the other internal rotators which will take some of the load off of infraspinatus/teres minor. Also, subscap can be stretched in the supine position.

The least invasive and easiest way to warm-up subscapularis is to place your finger pads on it while the arm is abducted and externally rotated, then adduct the arm by letting it lie in a comfortable position across your client's chest as shown in the photo below. This puts the muscle in a slack position (using the principle of positional release). Later on you'll take the humerus through a range of motion.

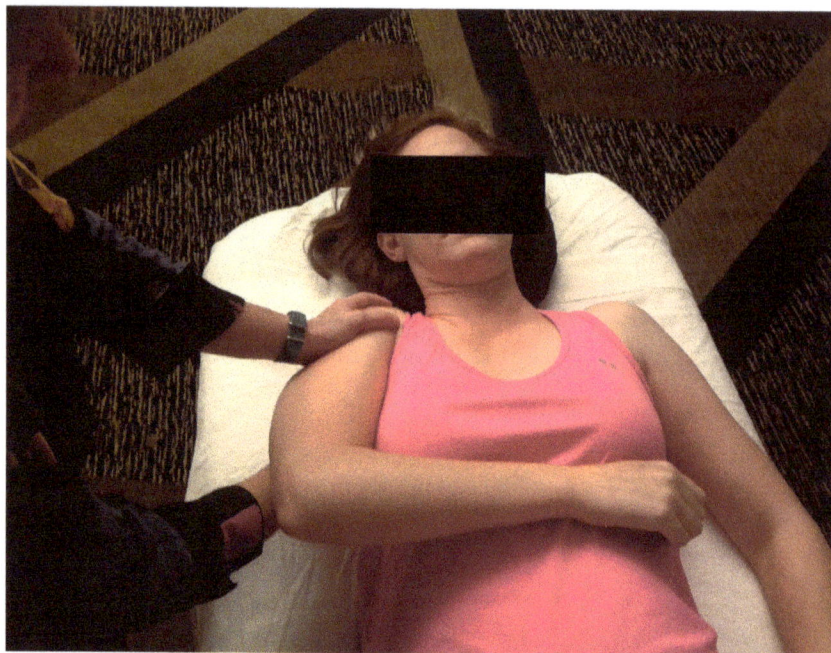

1.   A. Pin and Rock: Gently rock your client's shoulder while your fingers are gently pressing on subscapularis, working your way inferior to superior. Rocking is calming and a great way to "introduce" yourself to a muscle. The hand that is rocking the shoulder is the working hand. The hand that is on subscap is simply exerting a gentle pressure. Do this Pin and Rock until you feel some melting in the tissue. Perform it on as much of the subscap that is accessible. Notice if the scapula is glued on to the rib case. If it is, hopefully at the end of your work it will be more freely movable.

       B. Once you have felt some melting of the tissue you can add small circular movements of your finger tips as you continue to warm up the subscap. Do this with the muscle in a neutral state or if your client is too sore, a slacked state. Try to get as much length and width of subscapularis as you can.

There's been many clients on whom I could just do Step A for several sessions. "Unglueing" the subscapularis and freeing the scapula to glide on the thorax can take time. Honor your client's pain threshold. This builds rapport and trust.

2. Pin and Move: Take the shoulder through both passive and active range of motion while releasing trigger points and knots.

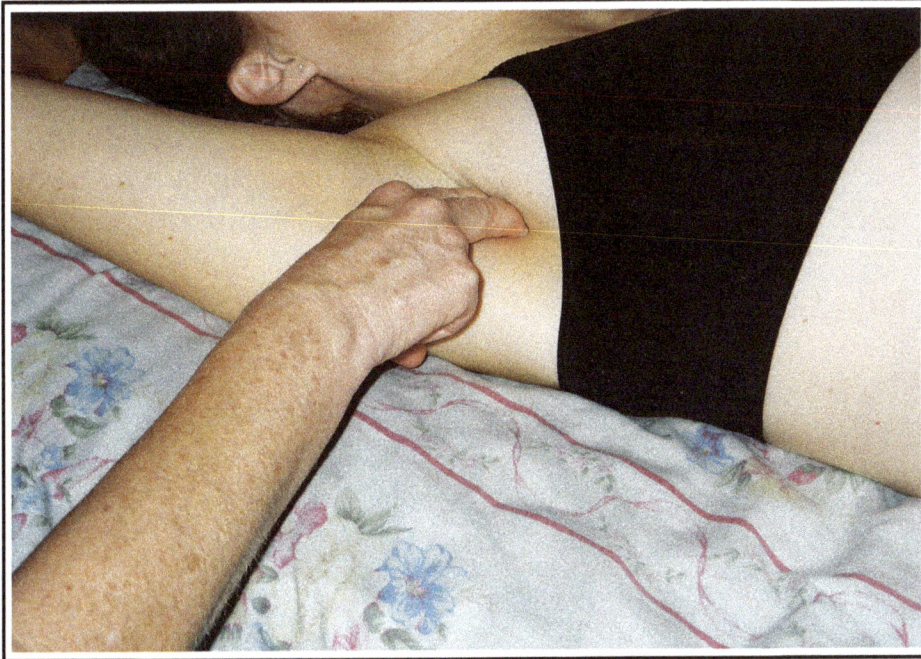

The photo above shows the client actively moving the humerus towards her ear in abduction while the therapist works the superior section of subscapularis in the supine position. Keep in mind that abduction is usually limited with rotator cuff injuries; work to increase range of movement while respecting limitations.

Active movement allows you to work through the muscle layers. Begin with passive movement to teach your client the movement pattern, then allow her to do it on her own. Keep in mind that most people with rotator cuff injuries have limited range of movement.

This active movement is essential for release of stubborn trigger points and knots.

MOVEMENT CHOICES:

- Internal and External rotation

- Abduction/adduction

- Any movement of the shoulder joint! You can always ask your client what movement she thinks would work.

27

3. **Releasing the tendon:** As you come to the superior section of the muscle, you'll find the subscapularis tendon by feeling for where the tissue thickens. On some people you'll be able to follow the tendon to its insertion on the lesser tubercle of the humerus. I suggest using your fingers (as shown in the photos) and not your thumbs. Keep your wrist in a neutral position as often as possible.

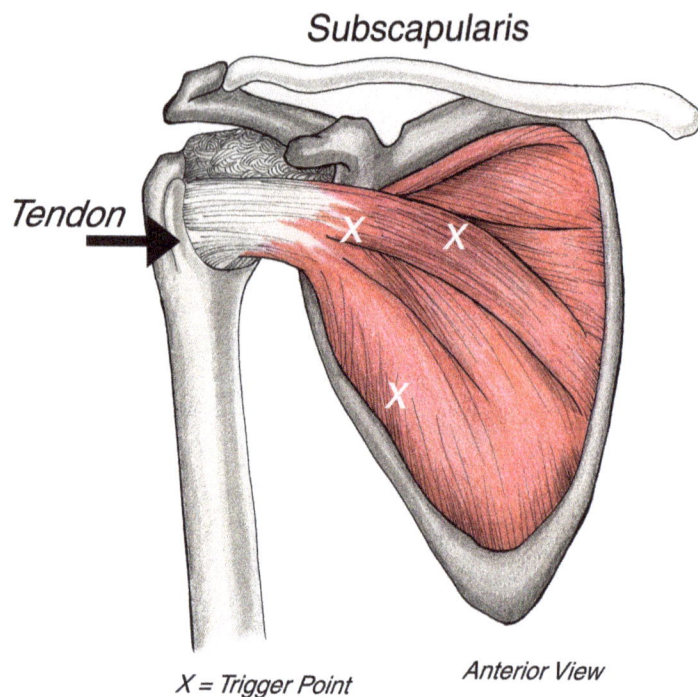

Subscapularis

Tendon ←

X = Trigger Point

Anterior View

Multi-directional fiber friction the tendon, modulating your pressure because this tissue can be quite tender. Do this in three positions:

A. Slack the muscle by internally rotating the humerus and add rocking to make this work less intense.

B. As the tissue softens, you can then move the shoulder joint into a neutral position and work the tendon.

C. Finally, multi-directional fiber friction the tendon with the joint externally rotated, putting the muscle in a stretched state.

Again, you may only be able to do Steps A and B or just Step A. Work with your client's pain tolerance. In many instances less is more!

4. **Releasing the tendons of infraspinatus/teres minor:** Before stretching the subscapularis, work the tendon of its antagonist: infraspinatus/teres minor. Often a client will have pain in the referral zone of the infraspinatus and teres minor while stretching the subscap. This is usually because those muscles have been eccentrically overloaded and fight against the subscap stretch.

To release infraspinatus and teres minor in the supine position, place your fingers up into the posterior crook of the shoulder joint on the posterior deltoid.

"Muscle swim" through posterior deltoid to get to the deeper layer of the infraspinatus and teres minor tendon. A medium pressure circular movement works well here. Use the weight of the client's arm for pressure.

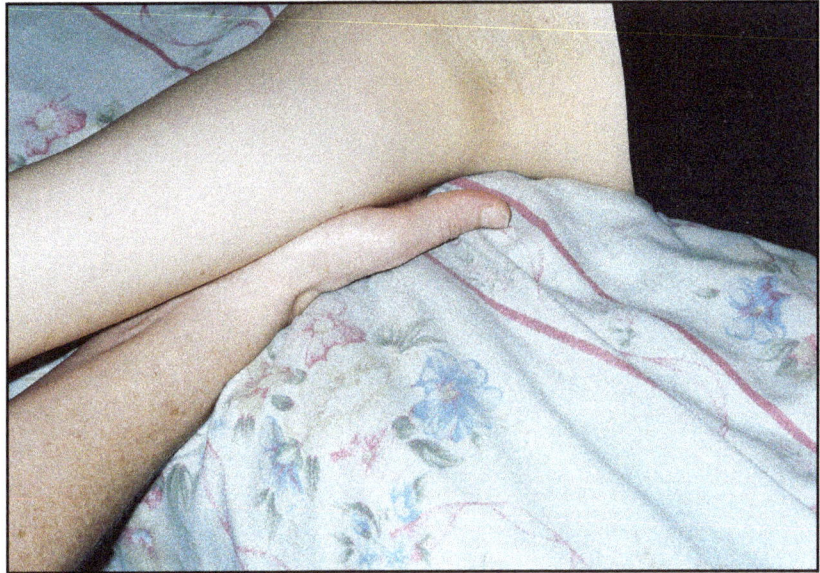

Working the tendons of infraspinatus and teres minor in the supine position.

Move the client's arm back and forth to create a multi-directional fiber friction and save your hands.

Traction the shoulder while working the tendons; hold the traction for about one minute with your fingers on the tendons.

Rocking is also a good technique to use here. I have found that gentle rocking encourages release of these overloaded tendons without forcing them into submission.

Once the tendons softens, slide your fingers medially to the belly of infraspinatus// teres minor. Use a medium pressure circular movement to warm up these muscles.

5. SUBSCAPULARIS STRETCH:

This muscle is usually locked short on most people, therefore stretching it along with the pectoralis major will help counteract a slumped, forward-shoulder posture. Instructions for stretching this muscle on a client with severely limited external rotation due to an injury or frozen shoulder is shown on the next page.

It's often necessary to release the muscle/tendon unit of subscap's antagonists, infraspinatus and teres minor, before doing this stretch because these eccentrically overloaded and locked long muscles fight against the subscap stretch. Make sure your client is feeling the stretch in the subscapularis or pectoralis major or latissimus dorsi/teres major which are other internal rotators of the humerus.

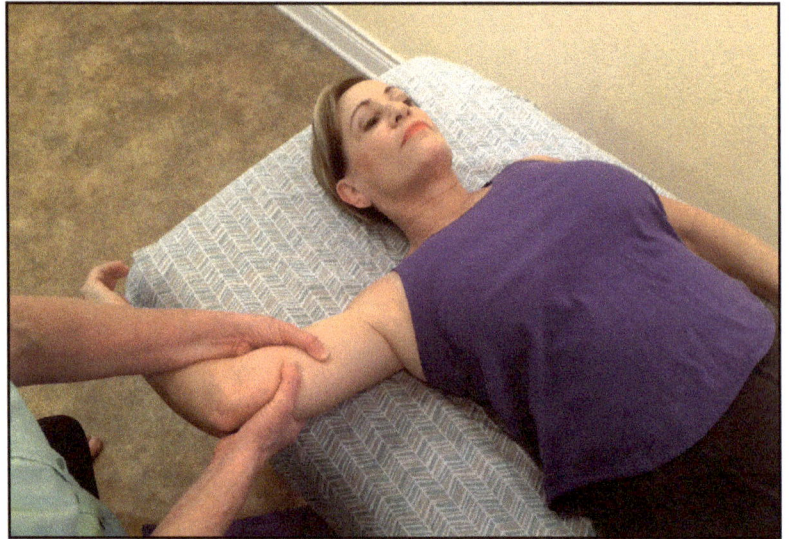

You can release the muscle/tendon unit of infraspinatus and teres minor by sliding your hand under your client's shoulder. The tendons of infraspinatus and teres minor are under posterior deltoid. Do some gentle circular massage on posterior deltoid to muscle swim to the deeper layer where the tendons of infraspinatus and teres minor live. Once you feel that tissue soften, slide your hand medially to warm up the belly of infraspinatus and teres minor. You may need to do this several times to get what I call a "clean stretch" - meaning that the sensation of stretch is felt in subscap or pectoralis major and/or latissimus dorsi/teres major. I highly recommend you use PNF (antagonist and agonist contract) techniques with this perennially locked short muscle.

A. Client is supine. With client's elbow bent, abduct the humerus to 90 degrees, traction and externally rotate the humerus. Gently push down on the forearm with your uphill forearm to slowly increase the external rotation of the humerus while maintaining the traction. Hold for 15-30 seconds.

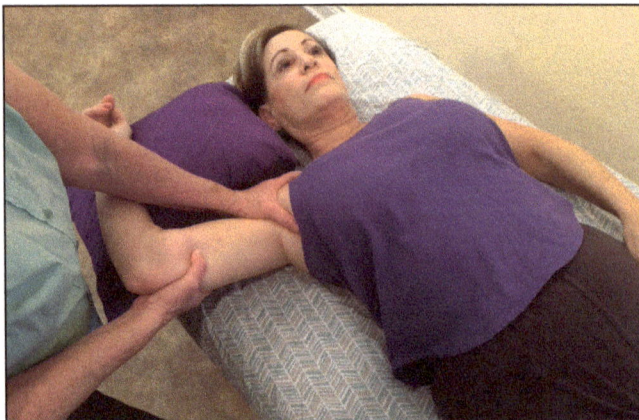

To stretch the subscap on a client with severely limited and painful external rotation due to an injury or frozen shoulder place a pillow or towel behind the arm to serve as a "boundary". Clients with painful external rotation are often quite guarded; the pillow reassures and protects them.

Stabilize the glenohumeral joint with your uphill hand while your downhill hand performs traction and external rotation.

Supine Subscapularis Protocols: The Short Version

Your mantra is: To accurately palpate subscap your fingers must be medial to the lateral border of the scapula!

1. **PIN AND ROCK:** Gently rock your client's shoulder and arm while your fingers are gently pressing on subscapularis. Begin with the muscle in a slack position, working your way inferior to superior. Repeat with the muscle in a neutral state and finally in a stretched state.

2. Continue to **warm up** the subscapularis using small circular movements of your fingers. Try and get as much length and width of the subscap as you can. Do this with the muscle in a neutral state or if your client is too sore, a slacked state.

3. **PIN AND MOVE/ TRIGGER POINT WORK:** Using one finger, start at the inferior portion of the muscle and search for trigger points. Ask your partner to help you identify those tender hot spots. When you find one, use active movement to release them. Internal/External rotation is a good starting movement. If Internal/External rotation does not produce significant change, try another movement pattern. You can add resistance to any movement pattern.

4. **MULTI-DIRECTIONAL FIBER FRICTION** the subscapularis tendon. Use rocking to save your hands!

5. **WARM-UP** the tendons of the infraspinatus and teres minor by "swimming" through posterior deltoid. Once they soften, slide your hand medially and warm up the belly of infraspinatus/ teres minor.

6. **Subscapularis stretch.**

IN THE SIDE-LYING POSITION:

You'll find that some clients will not be able to tolerate supine subscap work for a variety of reasons. They may be ticklish, have large breasts, be heavily muscled, or have a glued-down scapula that makes access to the subscap a challenge. Start those clients in the side-lying position.

Incorporate side-lying work with every client. Have your client roll on her side and place one arm on your shoulder. Position your hands as in the photo below. This is quite comfortable for both you and your client.

1. **Shoulder mobilizations:** The fingers of one hand pins the subscap while the other hand grasps the medial border of the scapula. Take the scapula through a range of motion: retraction, protraction, elevation, depression, upward and downward rotation. Dance with it! Mobilizations encourage and facilitate proper gliding of the scapula on the thorax.

2. **Trigger point work:** Using one finger, start at the inferior portion of the muscle and search for trigger points. You will most likely find some in this side-lying position that weren't apparent in supine. Ask your client to help you identify those tender hot spots. When you find one, use **active** movement to release them. You can add resistance to any movement pattern.

3. **Tendon work:** Multi-directional fiber friction the subscapularis tendon. Use rocking to save your hands!

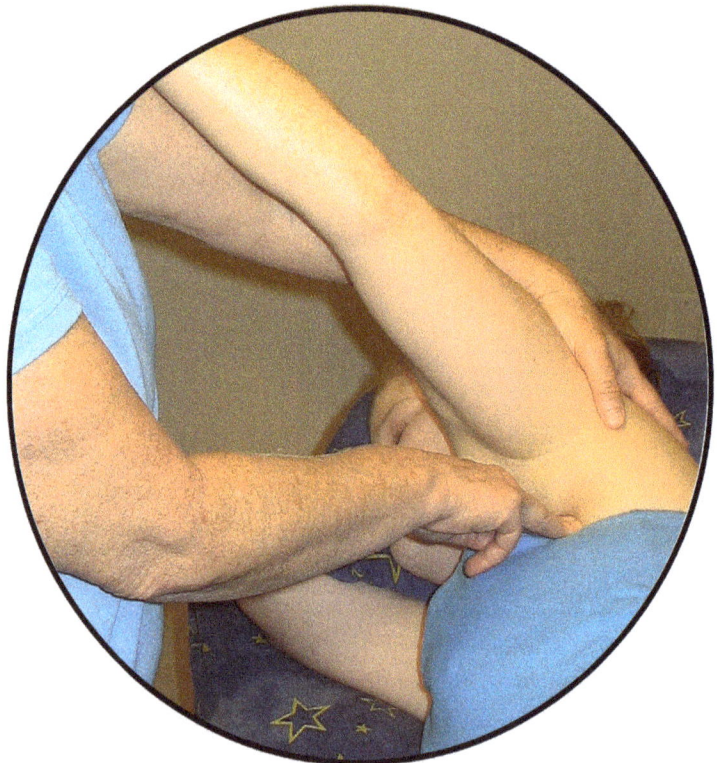

IN THE PRONE POSITION:

Find the lateral edge of latissimus dorsi and slide your fingers under it. Press your fingers pads up and you'll be on subscap.

1. **Shoulder mobilizations:** the fingers of one slide under latissimus to pin the subscap. Your other hand lifts the superior scapula. Take the scapula through a range of motion.

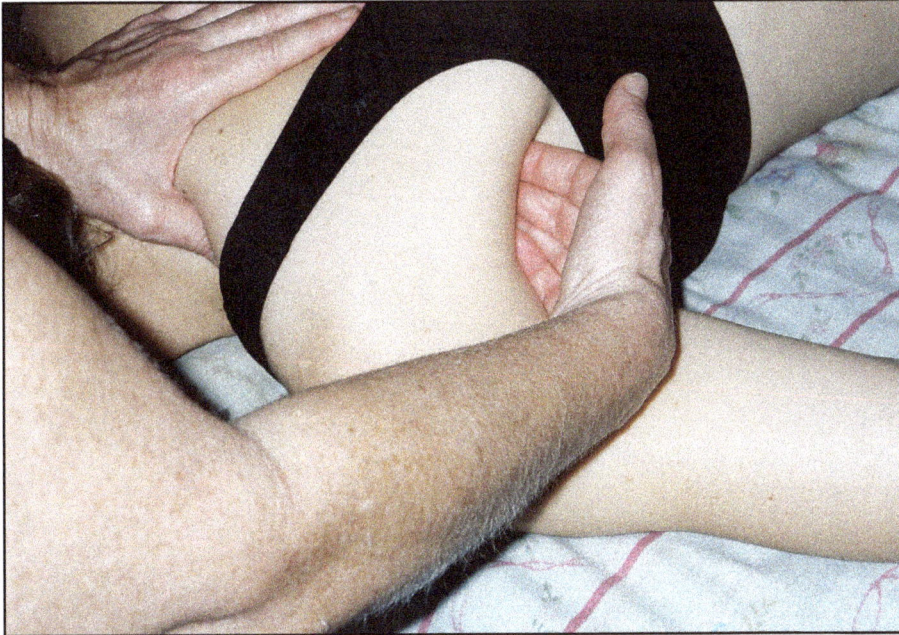

2. **Incorporate work on infraspinatus and supraspinatus.** In the photo left the therapist's right hand is working the subscapularis while her left thumb works the supraspinatus. This is an example of working two muscles at the same time.

•Educate the client about stretching this muscle (Broomstick stretch), sleeping position, and proper shoulder mechanics (see Client Education section).

INFRASPINATUS AND TERES MINOR MUSCLES

Actions: external rotation of the humerus at the shoulder joint and stabilization of the head of humerus in the glenoid fossa.

Attachments: medially to the infraspinous fossa on the scapula and laterally to the greater tubercle of the humerus.

The infraspinatus is a dense muscle with a thick fascial covering. The infraspinatus and teres minor blend into one tendon which unites with the shoulder joint capsule.

These muscles are almost always affected and have trigger points and most likely tendonitis or tendonosis. Clients will complain of pain "deep in the shoulder joint" and point to the front of their shoulder (anterior and medial deltoid). This pain in the deltoids is from trigger point referral. Trigger points also refer down the arm and sometimes to the posterior neck, suboccipitals and rhomboids/middle traps. It may be difficult to abduct or flex the humerus above the shoulder (180 degrees) since that requires a large degree of external rotation. It may also be difficult to completely internally rotate the humerus. Dysfunction of these muscles, as with any other rotator cuff muscle, will cause the other rotators to tighten up in an effort to compensate. Most of the time these muscles are overstretched (locked-long or held in an eccentric contraction) from their ongoing struggle with our overzealous internal rotators. These muscles are like David to the internal rotator's Goliath. Infraspinatus/teres minor aids in humeral depression as the humerus elevates. Weakness keeps humeral head in internal rotation thereby contributing to impingement syndrome as the greater tubercle is held in a anterior position.

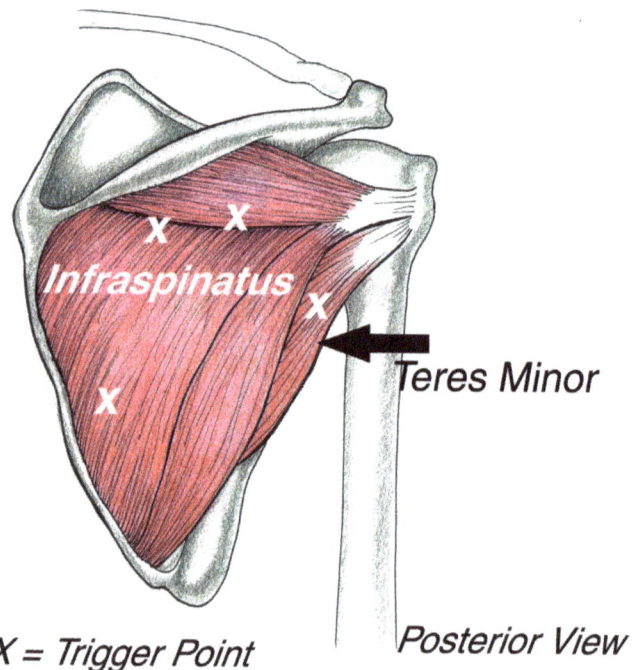

Trigger Point Patterns for Infraspinatus and Teres Minor

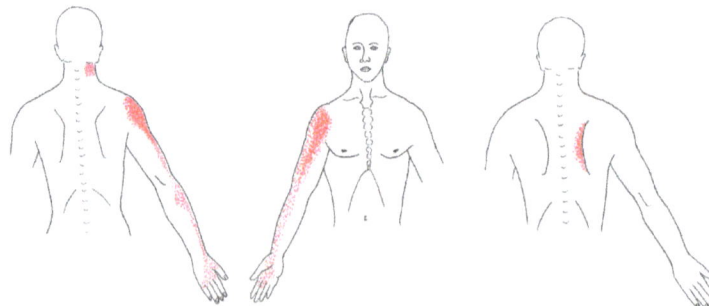

TECHNIQUES FOR WORKING THE INFRASPINATUS AND TERES MINOR

Work these muscles in all positions (supine, side-lying, or prone). You'll do most of your detail work in the prone position. You've already worked it supine during the subscapularis protocol. Include these muscles in your side-lying work. I give suggestions for side-lying strategies in this section.

The infraspinatus lies directly on the shoulder blade. The teres minor lies diagonally below and beside infraspinatus.

1. **Skin rolling:** We'll start by freeing the superficial fascia with skin rolling without lubricant in the prone position (photo right). Skin rolling helps to release the connective tissue (fascia). If you've already applied lubricant, simply wipe off with a towel. As you skin roll, feel for places where the skin won't give. Those are areas where the connective tissue is adhered or "glued" down. These areas will feel tender to your client. Gently work to unglue the areas.

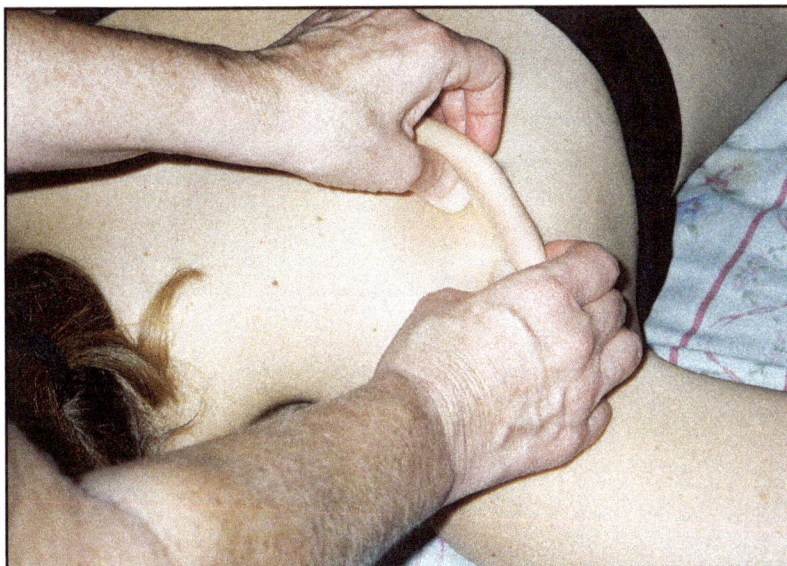

2. **Warm-up** the muscles with soothing gliding or kneading strokes.

3. **Muscle stripping:** Strip both muscles in a **lateral to medial direction** from and including the tendon to the medial attachments along the fiber orientation. This technique is sometimes referred to as *goading*. It's essential to go **lateral to medial** instead of medial to lateral because these muscles are locked long and need this goading to shorten and regain their contractibility.

Allow your fingers to "swim" gently and deeply through the tissue layers.

35

4. **Pin and Move:** Locate tender spots and trigger points and release with static compression and deep stroking over the point. *The photo below shows the therapist using her knuckle to release a trigger point in the prone position.*

Take the shoulder through both passive and active range of motion while working the tender spots and trigger points. Internal and external rotation is a good movement to begin with. Do the movement pattern passively for your client then have her do it **actively**. I like to use **active-resisted** movement on these muscles because the trigger points can be so entrenched. *

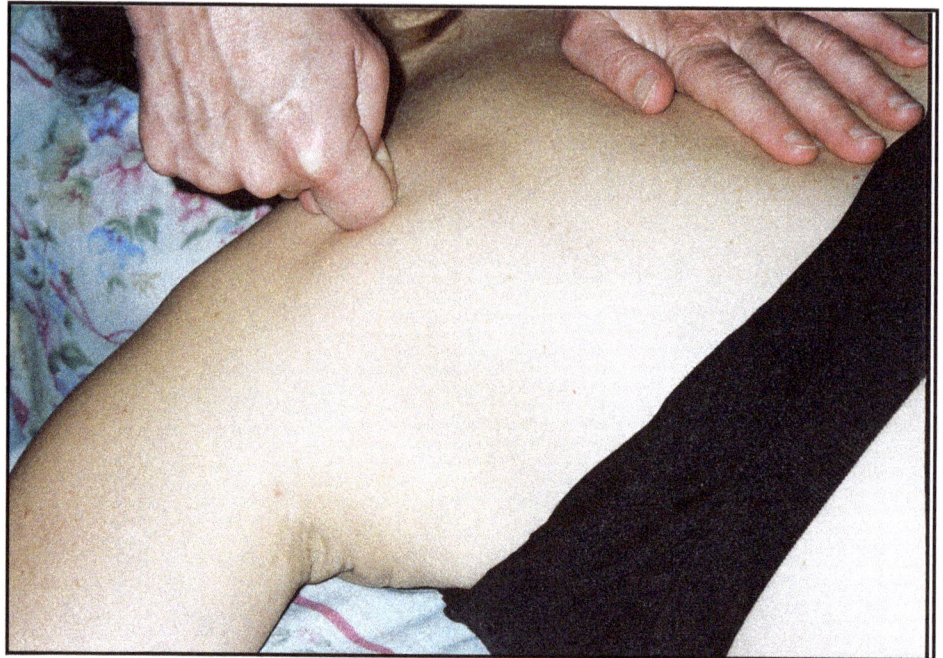

MOVEMENT CHOICES:

■ Internal and External rotation

■ Flexion/Extension

■ Any movement of the shoulder joint! I once was working on a client and having no success in clearing a trigger point. I finally remembered he was a golfer and had him swing his arm as if he was swinging a golf club, as best he could in the prone position. That was the magic movement and the trigger point released quite nicely.

■ Add resistance to any movement for especially stubborn trigger points and knots. I keep one pound and three pound weights under my table and put one in my client's hand if I need to recruit more muscle fibers with active-resisted movement. If you don't have weights, a can of soup will do! Or you can add resistance by having your client press into your hand or arm.

*Since infraspinatus/teres minor are usually locked long muscles, trigger points are actually serving a check-reigning function. It's as if groups of fibers have made an agreement to lock short to counterbalance the majority of locked long fibers. Hence, these trigger points are quite stubborn. Re-education of the muscles resting length with strength training is vital.

5. Releasing the tendons of infraspinatus/teres minor: Be sure to work the tendons, which can be quite sensitive and full of adhesions.

The infraspinatus and teres minor blend into one co-joint thick and sturdy tendon which unites with the joint capsule. The tendons terminate on the greater tubercle of the humerus.

Multi-directional fiber friction is excellent for reducing and preventing scar tissue formation. I like to use a small hot stone for this work.

To save your hands, alternate moving the humerus with moving your hands. Both create a good cross-fiber friction.

Using a small heated stone for your multi-directional friction also saves your hands and melts the tissue beautifully.

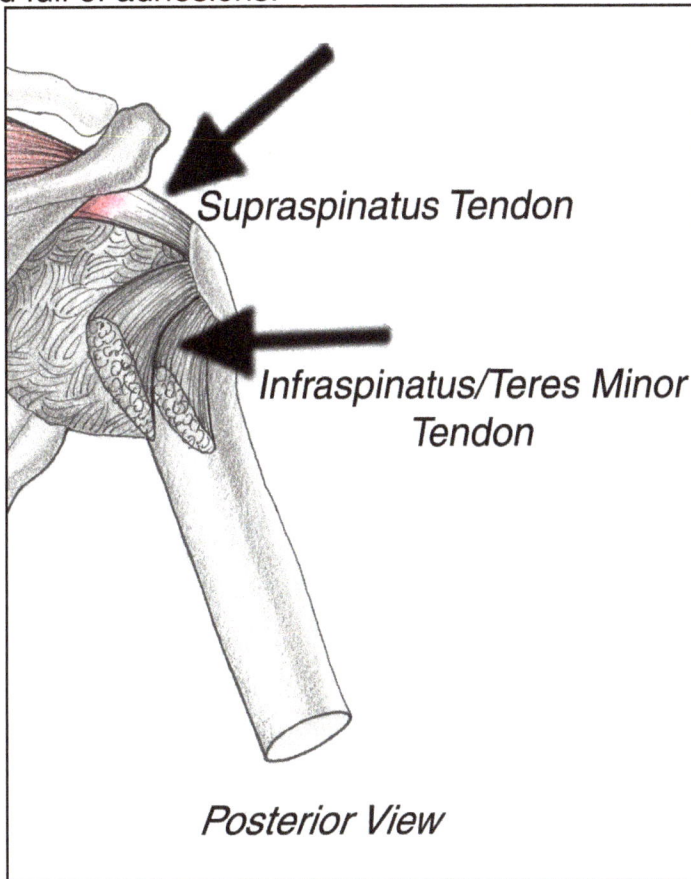

Supraspinatus Tendon

Infraspinatus/Teres Minor Tendon

Posterior View

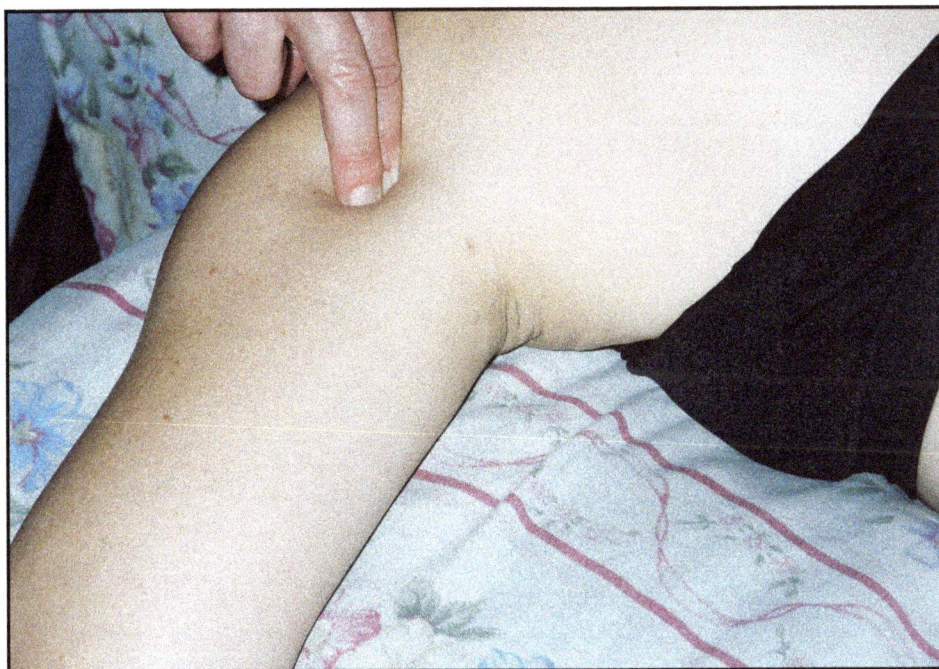

Multi-directional friction on the tendons in the prone position.

37

6. **Vibration:** Use a fast paced spindle-stimulating technique such as vibration over both muscles to help tone these weak, inhibited muscles. The muscle spindle governs the stretch reflex which is a neuro-muscular reaction that involves an involuntary contraction, or spasm, of a muscle subjected to a pulling force.

7. End with a calming effleurage to say "goodbye."

8. Remember, you can incorporate working the other rotator cuff muscles while doing this infraspinatus/teres minor work.

9. This is a good opportunity to address the rhomboids and middle traps. These muscles are in the infraspinatus referral zone and are likely candidates for developing their own trigger points. A round shouldered posture will cause these muscles to become locked long and unable to fulfill their duties as stabilizers of the scapulae. The suggested protocols for infraspinatus/teres minor work well for rhomboids and middle traps.

10. Do *not* stretch these muscles, as they are probably overstretched. Educate the client about strengthening these muscles, sleeping position, and proper shoulder mechanics (see Client Education section).

PRONE INFRASPINATUS/TERES MINOR PROTOCOLS:
THE SHORT VERSION

1. **SKIN ROLLING** (no lubricant): Cover the entire area, including supraspinatus, upper traps, rhomboids and middle traps.

2. **WARM-UP** the muscles with a soothing petrissage. A one-handed petrissage works best on these small muscles.

3. **STRIP** both muscles in a lateral to medial direction from and including the tendon to the medial attachments along the fiber orientation. This technique is sometimes referred to as goading.

4. **PIN AND MOVE/ TRIGGER POINT WORK:** Locate tender spots and trigger points and release with static compression and deep stroking over the point. Use active movement to release the points. Internal/external rotation is a good choice here.

5. **MULTI-DIRECTIONAL FIBER** friction the tendons.

6. **FAST PACED SPINDLE-STIMULATING VIBRATION** to help tone these weak, inhibited muscles.

7. **END** with a calming effleurage to say "goodbye."

IN THE SIDE-LYING POSITION:
Position your client as you would for side-lying subscapularis.

1. **Strip** both muscles in a **lateral to medial direction** from and including the tendon to the medial attachments along the fiber orientation. This technique is sometimes referred to as goading.

2. **Trigger point work:** Locate tender spots and trigger points and release with static compression and deep stroking over the point. You will most likely find some in this side-lying position that weren't apparent in the prone position. Use **active** movement to release the points.

SUPRASPINATUS MUSCLE

Actions: abduction of the humerus at the shoulder joint and stabilization of the head of humerus in the glenoid fossa.

Attachments: medially to the supraspinatus fossa and laterally to the greater tubercle of the humerus.

The supraspinatus is the most active rotator cuff muscle. It's also the most frequently torn rotator cuff muscle because of its location. The junction of the muscle belly and tendon is susceptible to chronic tearing of fibers from impingement underneath the acromion process. *(See **Figure F** on page 12.)* These chronic tears will frequently develop into long-term problems of chronic pain and loss of range of motion. The supraspinatus tendon joins with the tendon of the infraspinatus and teres minor to form an expansive domelike tendon that blends with the joint capsule. This muscle can mimic bursitis if it has trigger points; pain will be felt in the deltoid region down to the elbow. Trigger points can also refer to the subocciptal region. Carrying a heavy object with the arms extended can cause trigger points, since the supraspinatus has to work very hard to prevent downward dislocation of the head of the humerus. For a client who has severe dysfunction in this muscle, even swinging the arms while walking can be painful.

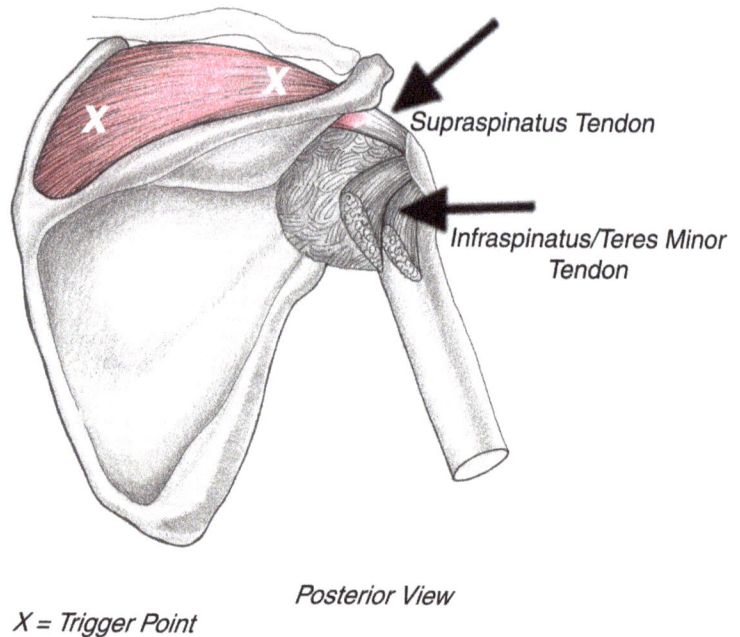

Supraspinatus Tendon

Infraspinatus/Teres Minor Tendon

Posterior View

X = Trigger Point

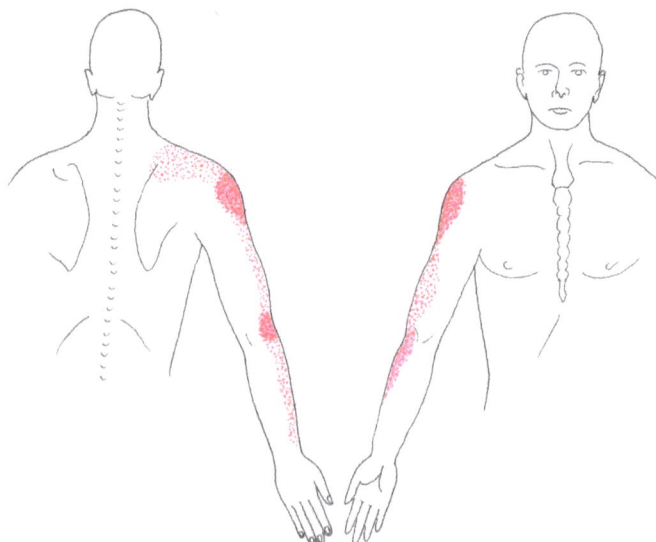

Trigger Point Patterns for Supraspinatus

TECHNIQUES FOR WORKING THE SUPRASPINATUS

Work this muscle in all positions (supine, side-lying, or prone). I generally do most of my detailed work in the side-lying position and it's the best position to stretch the supraspinatus. Include deep gliding strokes on supraspinatus during your supine and prone work.

The supraspinatus lies directly on top of the shoulder blade in the supraspinatus fossa, posterior and under the trapezius. Push the trapezius anterior and you'll find the small, but meaty supraspinatus muscle. **Move superior even a centimeter and you're off supraspinatus and on trapezius. You should always feel the ledge of the spine of the scapula to ensure you are precisely on the supraspinatus.**

IN THE SIDE-LYING POSITION:

1. **Skin Rolling:** We'll start by freeing the superficial fascia with skin rolling without lubricant.

2. **Warm-up:** After your skin rolling, with a small amount of lubricant, warm-up the muscle by gliding your fingers **medial to lateral** with firm but tolerable pressure. It may take some time to get through the constricted and tense upper traps; be patient.

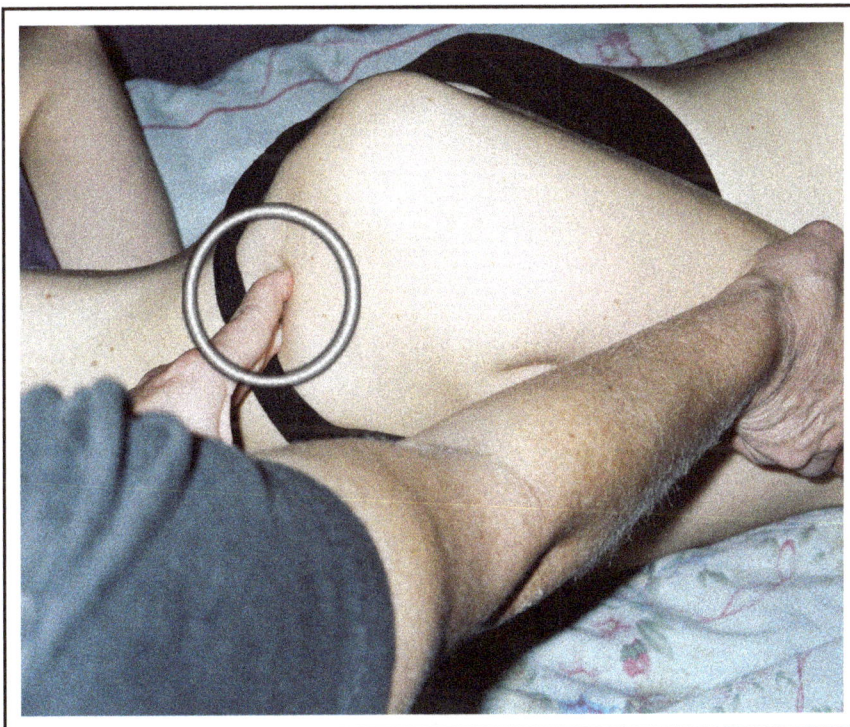

Working the supraspinatus in the side-lying position. Notice that the therapist's fingers are in the supraspinatus fossa.

41

3. **Tendon work:** The supraspinatus tendon dives under the acromion. This area can be extremely tender and full of adhesions. If your client reports unbearable or exquisite pain, there may be bursitis. If you suspect bursitis, simply omit this step and refer to a doctor. Bursitis can take time to resolve; it responds well to ultrasound. You and your client should always keep in mind the question: *What caused the bursitis and how can the client change her shoulder mechanics to eliminate the perpetuating factors?*

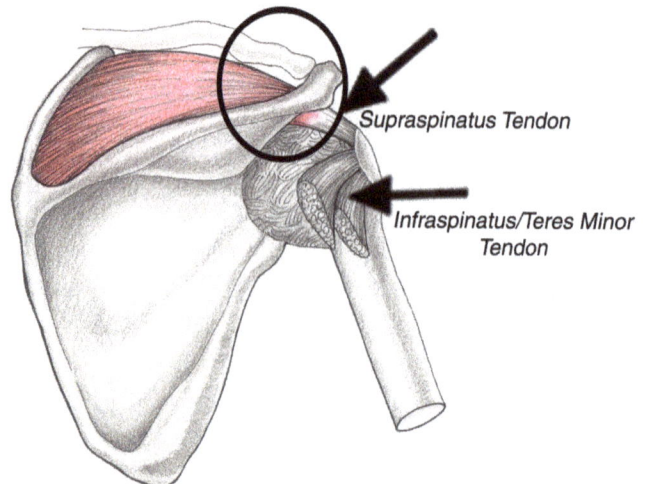

Supraspinatus Tendon

Infraspinatus/Teres Minor Tendon

Posterior View

Work the tendon as far laterally as possible, moving your fingers anterior to posterior using **multi-directional fiber friction**. Include the attachment on the greater tubercle.

4. **Pin and Move:** When the muscle is warm locate any taut bands and trigger points and release with static pressure. Take the shoulder through both passive and **active** range of motion while working the trigger points. If your client reports a trigger point referral that wraps around the side of the temple, this is a classic trapezius referral pattern. This means you are not quite down to the supraspinatus layer. Work to release this point which should then allow you to access the deeper supraspinatus.

MOVEMENT CHOICES:

■ Abduction/Adduction

■ Flexion/Extension

■ Any movement of the shoulder joint!

■ Add resistance to any movement for especially stubborn trigger points and knots. I keep one pound and three pound weights under my table and put one in my client's hand if I need to recruit more muscle fibers with active-resisted movement. If you don't have weights, a can of soup will do! Or you can add resistance by having your client press into your hand or arm.

This is a good opportunity to also massage the medial deltoid, which is lateral to the supraspinatus.

5. Say "goodbye" to the supraspinatus with some calming effleurage strokes. Follow this with the stretch below.

6. SIDE-LYING STRETCH OF THE SUPRASPINATUS:

One hand presses the shoulder towards the client's hips while the other hand tractions and presses the humerus behind the back in adduction. If the client is feeling too much stretch in the neck and not enough in the supraspinatus, have her bend her elbow and place a pillow under the head.

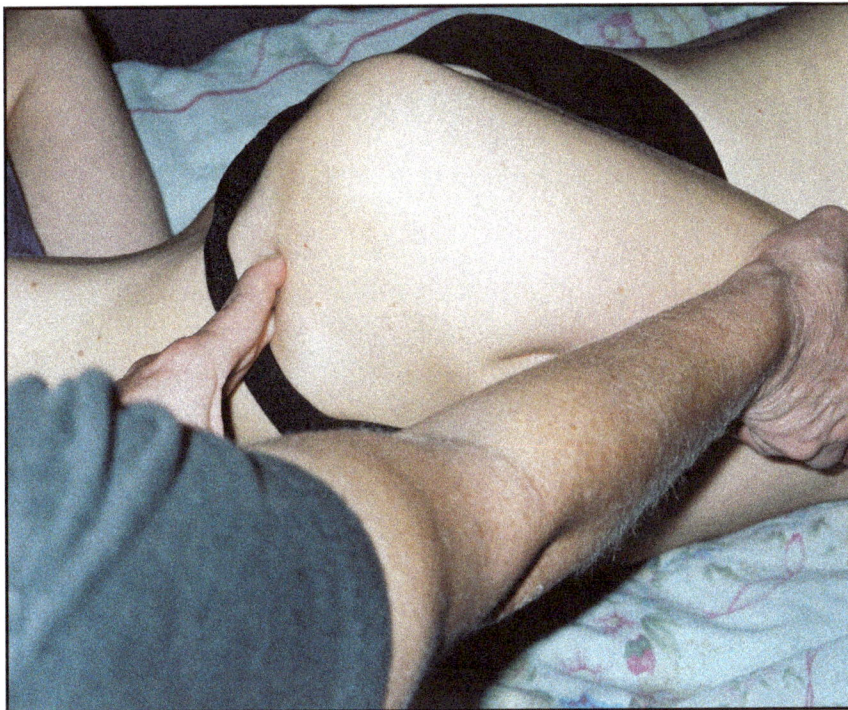

Pinning the supraspinatus while you stretch it *(shown left)* can facilitate the stretch and allow the client to differentiate between the sensation of stretch in the supraspinatus and the neck.

Include working the supraspinatus in your prone work also!

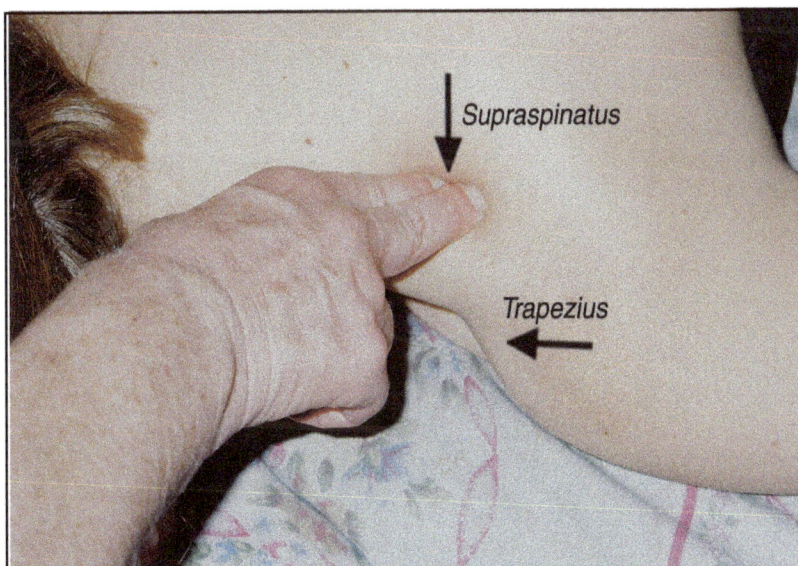

Working the supraspinatus in the prone position.

Educate the client about stretching this muscle and proper shoulder mechanics (see Client Education section).

SIDE-LYING SUPRASPINATUS PROTOCOLS:
THE SHORT VERSION

1. **SKIN ROLL** supraspinatus - no lubricant.

2. **STRIP** supraspinatus in a medial to lateral direction to encourage lengthening.

3. **MULTI-DIRECTIONAL fiber friction** the area where the muscle dives under the acromion process.

4. **MULTI-DIRECTIONAL fiber friction** the attachment at the greater tubercle.

5. **PIN AND MOVE/TRIGGER POINT WORK:** search out and release trigger points. Use active movement to release the points. Abduction/Adduction is a good movement to start with.

6. **CALMING EFFLEURAGE** to "say goodbye"

7. **SUPRASPINATUS STRETCH.**

LONG HEAD OF BICEPS TENDON

Actions: the long head of the biceps draws the head of the humerus upward into the glenoid fossa and helps stabilize the shoulder joint.
Attachment: glenoid labrum of the scapula.

The biceps does more than flex the elbow. The long head of the biceps is considered the "fifth rotator cuff" because of its stabilizing influence on the humerus and scapula. It's located between the supraspinatus tendon on the greater tubercle and subscapularis tendon on the lesser tubercle, in the bicipital groove. The long head also is a major decelerator of the throwing arm. It's effectiveness as a stabilizer is dependent on it's proper position in the groove and rotator cuff injuries can affect its positioning. Tendonitis, or, more precisely tenosynovitis, of the long head of the biceps often accompanies rotator cuff injuries. The groove that it sits in can be narrow, and repeated movements of the shoulder can cause the tendon and its synovial sheath to rub against either the lesser or greater tubercles, causing micro-tearing. The supraspinatus tendon, long head of the biceps, and the subacromial bursa are close neighbors, and inflammation of any of these structures may cause them to take up more valuable space, resulting in impingement, which results in more inflammation, etc. Pulling exercises that require the humerus to move against resistance can aggravate this condition. It's important to note that pain from tenosynovitis of the long head is in the referral zone of both supraspinatus and infraspinatus and could be mistaken for trigger point referral. Always check this structure to see if it's painful.

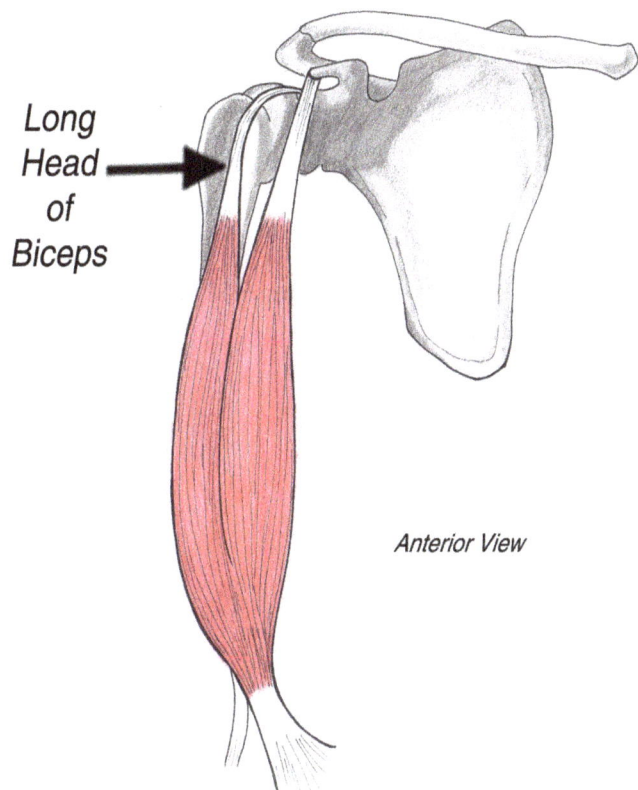

Long Head of Biceps

Anterior View

TECHNIQUES FOR WORKING THE LONG HEAD OF THE BICEPS

To find the long head of the biceps, position the arm in neutral and place your thumb on the head of the humerus. Rotate the arm back and forth, looking for a groove between two bumps (the greater and lesser tubercles). When you find the groove, you'll be on the long head of the biceps.

1. **Skin Rolling:** Begin by skin rolling (without lubricant) over the entire shoulder area to release the connective tissue. If you've already applied lubricant, simply wipe off with a towel. As you skin roll, feel for places where the skin won't give. Those are areas where the connective tissue is adhered or "glued" down. These areas will feel tender to your client. Gently work to unglue the areas.

2. **Pin and Move:** Search for trigger points in the belly of the biceps and apply static pressure to them. These trigger points are generally created by pain referral from the infraspinatus muscle.

3. **Tendon Work:** Multi-directional fiber friction the tendon, *(photo right),* looking for areas of maximum tenderness. Keep your movements small, as you can dislodge the tendon. Work within the client's pain threshold. Icing this tendon along with the tendons of the supraspinatus, infraspinatus, and teres minor helps reduce inflammation and soreness.

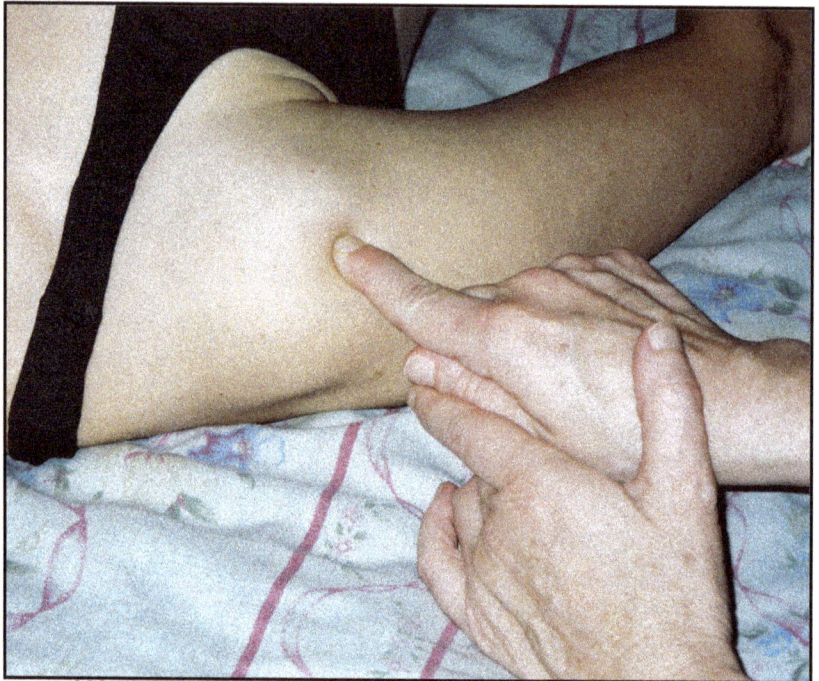

Working the long head of the biceps in the supine position.

•Educate the client about proper shoulder mechanics (see Client Education section).

•Instruct your clients to cross-fiber their own long head of the biceps!

Feel before acting and follow the cues of the client.

PECTORALIS MAJOR MUSCLE

Actions: flexion, extension, adduction, and internal rotation of the humerus.
Attachments: medially to the clavicle, sternum, and costal fibers of ribs 2-7; laterally to the crest of the greater tubercle of the humerus.

This muscle exerts a powerful internal rotation on the humerus, is usually locked short and must be released and stretched in order to correct rotator cuff injuries. Many people overwork their pecs and neglect their upper back muscles. A client who is experiencing a rotator cuff problem would be well advised to decrease his strengthening of the pectoralis major and stretch it more often. A habitually slumped, round-shouldered, head-forward posture will shorten the pec major. As with all of these muscles, correct posture is paramount to complete recovery.

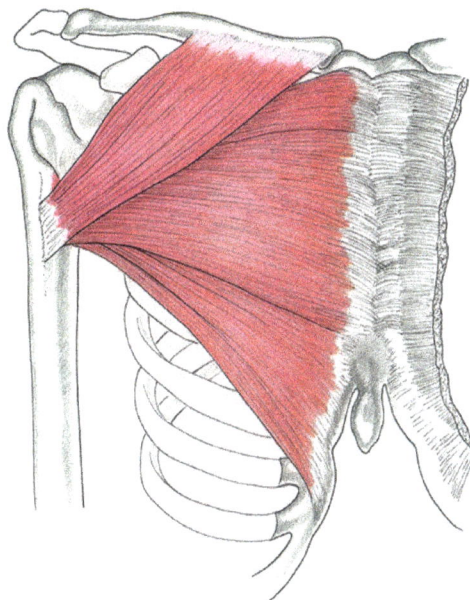

TECHNIQUES FOR WORKING THE PECTORALIS MAJOR

1. **Warm-Up:** Client is supine. Warm up the muscle with effleruage and petrissage. Increase length by gliding the fingers **medial to lateral** with firm but tolerable pressure. Working across the client's body *(shown in photo right)* allows the therapist more range of motion. Work to elongate the muscle from its medial attachments on the sternum, clavicle, and costal cartilage out to its lateral attachment on the bicipital groove of the humerus. To facilitate the release of the connective tissue, use only a small amount of lubricant, if any.

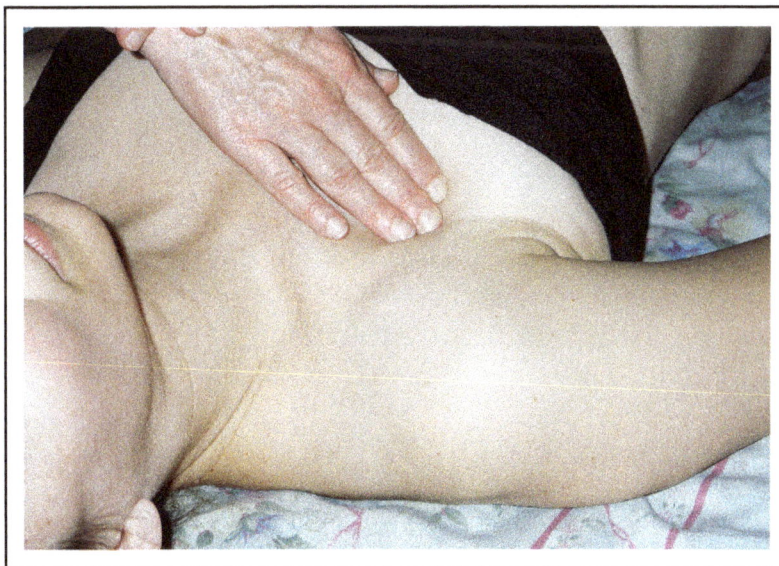

Working the pec with the client's arm at her side.

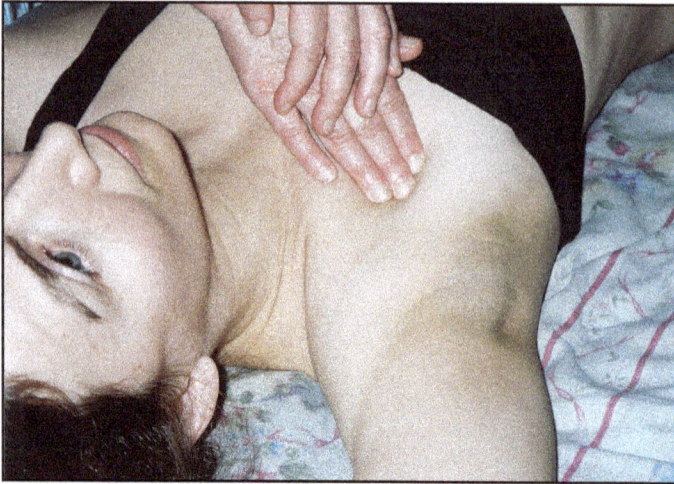

Working the pec major towards the tendon with the client sliding her arm towards her ear (abduction/adduction.)

2. **Pin and Move:** Take the arm through active range of motion while working the muscle:

A.) Abduction and adduction
B.) Internal and external rotation.

Have your client turn her head away from the side you are working as she moves her arm. This helps to lengthen pec major. Take this opportunity to massage the anterior deltoid which is lateral to the pectoralis major and which also internally rotates the shoulder joint. End with a "goodbye" effleurage.

3. SUPINE STRETCH FOR THE PECTORALIS MAJOR:
Have client move close to the side of the table of the arm to be stretched.
A. Abduct the arm to about 90° and externally rotate the shoulder. Gently traction and press the humerus and forearm down.

B. Abduct the arm slightly higher, maintaining external rotation and traction, and press down again. Repeat this (abducting the arm slightly higher and higher, pressing down and holding) until the arm is in flexion.

To make the stretch *less* intense, bend the elbow and do not press on the forearm; only press on the humerus. If numbness and tingling in the forearm and fingers occur, it may be an indication of thoracic outlet syndrome. Thoracic outlet syndrome is a compression of the brachial plexus and/or the axillary vessels which can have several causes, including brachial plexus impingement by pectoralis minor and/or scalenes. Decreasing the intensity of the stretch will usually ease the symptoms. Release of the scalenes is beyond the scope of this book; the pectoralis minor is discussed in the next section.

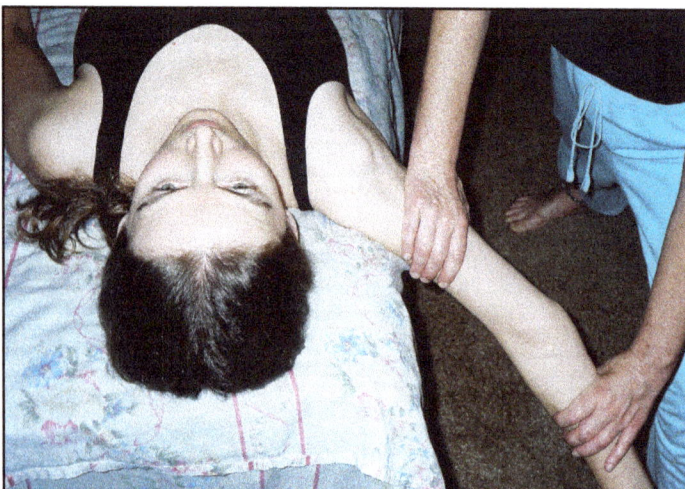

A.

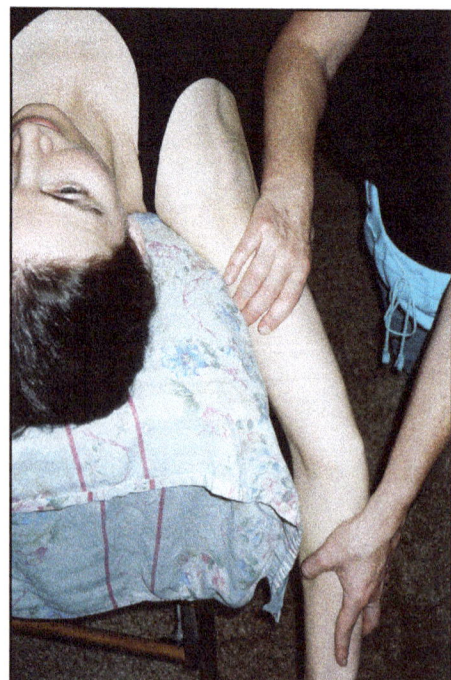

B.

4. ALTERNATE STRETCHES FOR THE PECTORALIS MAJOR AND INTERNAL ROTATORS USING A BALL OR PILLOWS:

A. Using about a 12-inch diameter soft ball, have the client sit up and place the ball covered with a pillow case or towel in the mid-thoracic region. In the *photo right* the ball is not covered for better visibility. Support the client's neck and have her slowly lie back over the ball.

Gently let the head and neck down. Some clients may need the extra support of a pillow under the head/neck. Every client is different, so sometimes it's necessary to play with the placement of the ball (either higher or lower) to get the right "fit."

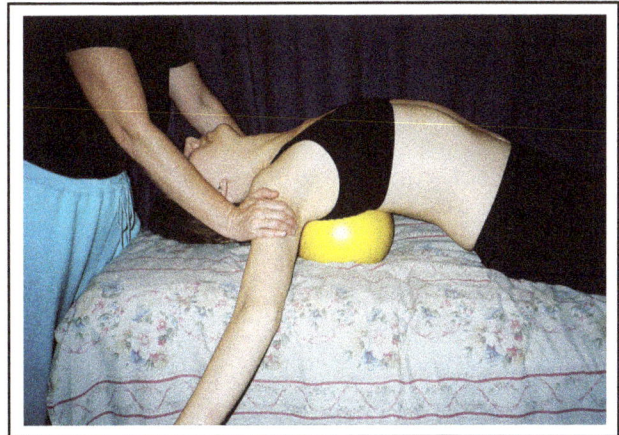

A

Once the client is situated, press down on each humerus to open the area. Encourage your client to breathe deeply during this stretch. If the client experiences any lower back pain, try having the client bend her knees. If that doesn't work, discontinue the stretch or try a smaller ball. This is also a wonderful stretch for the sternocleidomastoid and scalenes (make sure you warm them up before stretching). Clients can be encouraged to do this as a self-stretch.

B. Client is supine. Prop one or two pillows under the client's mid-back so the head is in hyperextension, yet supported by the table. The number of pillows and the placement of the arms depends on the flexibility of your client. For a client with limited flexibility, start with one pillow with the arms out to the side. **Make sure the shoulders are externally rotated.** Gently press the upper arms down toward the table. This stretch is also great for deepening the breath.

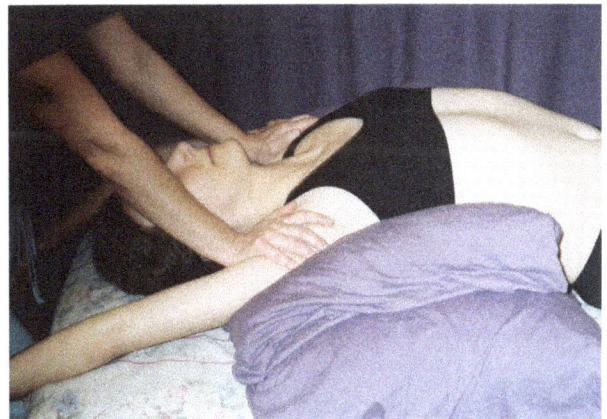

Your client will also be getting a gentle sternocleidomastoid stretch (make sure you warm that muscle up before stretching). You can massage the lower body while the client enjoys this stretch. Clients can be encouraged to do this as a self-stretch.

B

5. Educate the client about stretching this muscle and proper shoulder mechanics (see Client Education section).

───────────●───────────

PECTORALIS MINOR MUSCLE

Actions: depresses and protracts the scapula and assists in forced inspiration.
Attachments: superior - coracoid process of the scapula; inferior - near the costal fibers of ribs 3-5.

A tight pectoralis minor will pull the shoulder blade anterior and inferior, taking the head of the humerus with it, thus preventing the rotator cuff from working effectively by shortening the internal rotators and placing the external rotators in a locked long position. A shortened pec minor also restricts scapular movement. I have found that many rotator cuff dysfunctions begin with a tight pec minor. You can spot a tight pec minor in a client by having her lie in the supine position; look for the shoulder that is more anterior. Tight internal rotators can also cause this and the two often go hand in hand. A tight pectoralis minor can also impinge the axillary artery and brachial plexus, causing numbness in the ulnar side of the forearm, hand, or fingers. Trigger points refer to the front of the chest and shoulder and the ulnar side of the arm and fingers. A habitually slumped, round-shouldered, head-forward posture will shorten the pec minor as will chest breathing and repetitive, forceful downward motions of the arms. The muscle must be released and stretched for the scapula to find it's normal resting place and to allow the rotator cuff to work effectively.

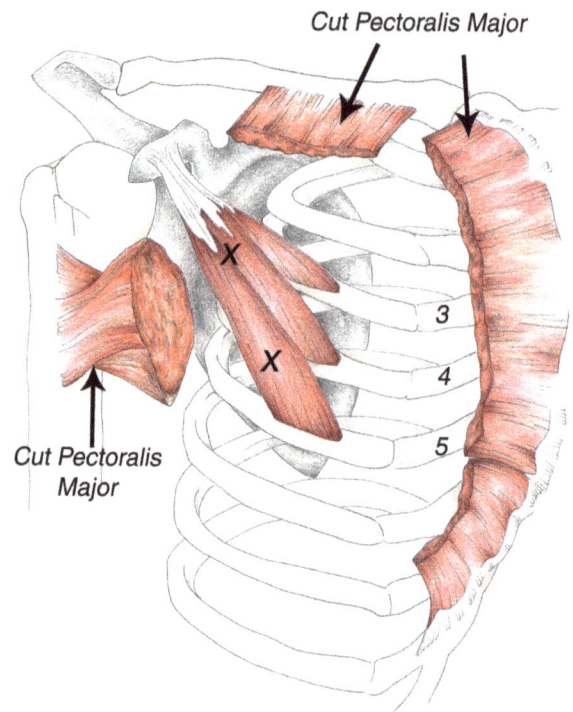

Cut Pectoralis Major

Cut Pectoralis Major

TECHNIQUES FOR WORKING THE PECTORALIS MINOR

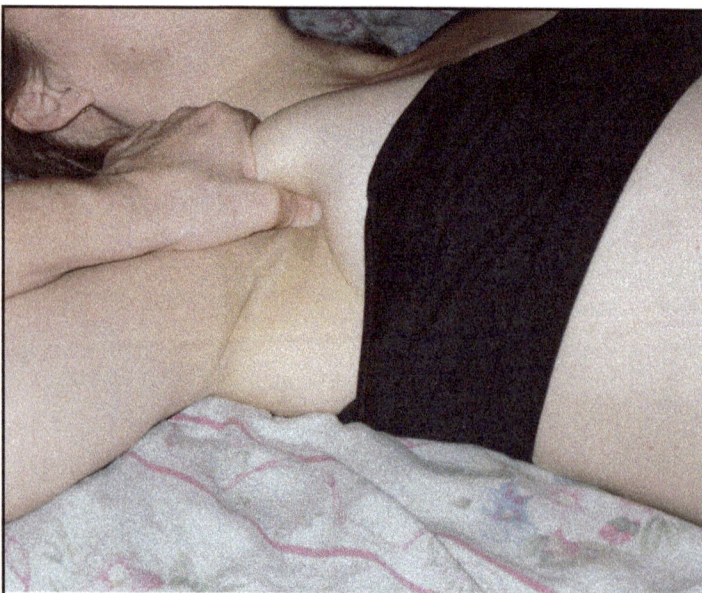

Work the obstinate pec minor in both the supine and side-lying positions. I like to begin my work on pec minor in the supine position after I've done my work on pec major. You can access the pec minor by pushing your thumb in *under* pec major from the client's side *(photo left)*. Feel for a diagonal band of tissue.

1. **Pin and Rock:** This muscle can be quite tender, so work within your client's pain threshold. Use the pin and rock technique to soften and prepare pec minor for deeper work. Gently pin pec minor anywhere on the belly and rock your client's shoulder.

2. **Longitudinal stripping:** When you feel the muscle relax a bit, begin longitudinal stripping from the attachments at the ribs to the attachment at the coracoid process. Stroking in this direction encourages the muscle to lengthen. As you work to release the pec minor, place your other hand under your client's back and passively move the scapula in towards the spine and away from the spine in retraction and protraction. If your client finds this work to be too painful, you can hold the scapula in protraction while you work, which puts in the muscle in a slack position. I have found that massaging it, then stretching it, then massaging it again to be effective, as pec minor can be difficult to release.

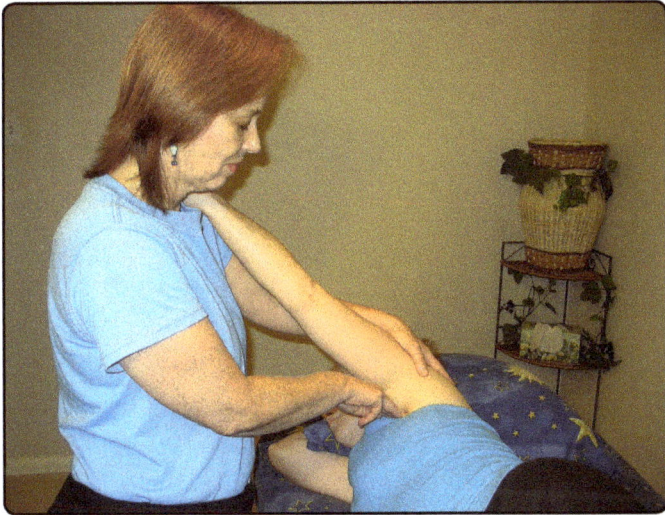

3. This muscle needs all the help it can get to release so I always include side-lying work. Place the client's hand on your shoulder and stabilize the scapula with that hand. You can then slide the fingers of your other hand under pec major and feel for the diagonal band of pec minor. Rocking and deep longitudinal stripping are good choice here as well. As always, include passive and active movement. **Active retraction and protraction of the scapula are good choices here.**

4. PEC MINOR STRETCH:

Client is side-lying. Abduct the humerus 180°, externally rotate the shoulder joint, then elevate and retract the scapula. The arrow pointing *down* refers to the retraction of the scapula. The arrow pointing *left* refers to the elevation of the scapula. Make sure the client's lower back does not fall backward or forward.

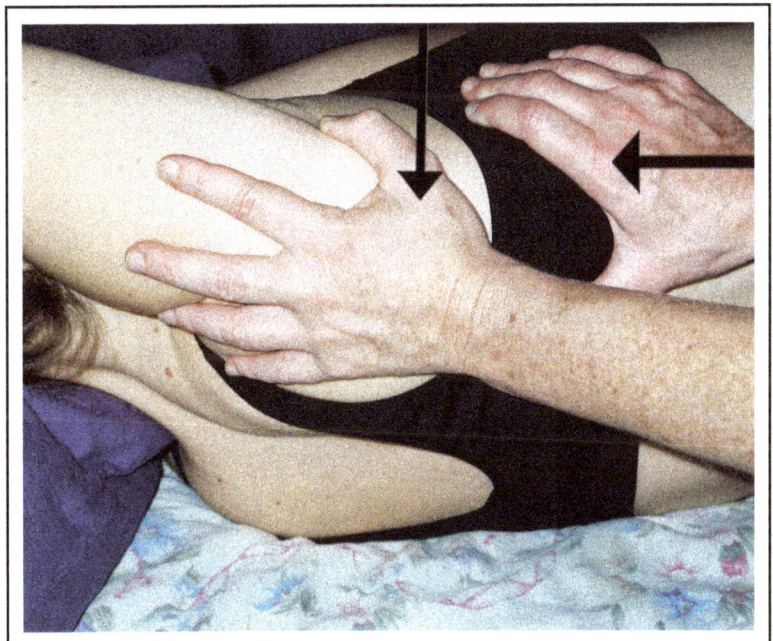

Stretching the right pectoralis minor

SERRATUS ANTERIOR MUSCLE

Actions: protracts and upwardly rotates the scapula and prevents "winging" of the scapula. Attachments: anterior - superior lateral surfaces of upper eight or nine ribs; posterior - anterior surface of the medial border of scapula.

The serratus anterior is an important muscle for shoulder girdle stabilization torso alignment. When it's locked short it pulls the scapula, shoulder, head, and neck forward and restricts the lateral movement of the ribs in respiration because it's usually locked onto the costal attachments. Since the serratus and the trapezius upwardly rotate the scapula, a tight serratus can limit abduction of the humerus above 60 degrees. The humerus cannot rise above 60 degrees of abduction unless the acromion process of the scapula is lifted out of the way of the humerus. Tightness in the serratus can also make it difficult to reach back or pull your shoulder blades together. Its fan-shaped fiber direction provides its ability to move the scapulae in different planes.

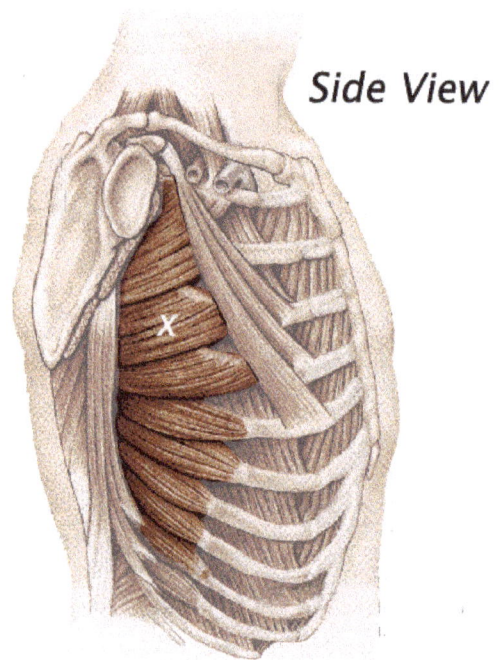

Side View

Trigger points in the serratus anterior refer to the lower medial border of the scapula, along the lateral ribs, and down the ulnar side of the arm. Travell calls it the "stitch in the side" muscle because trigger points can be activated by deep breathing since it assists expansion of the ribs when you need more air, or high levels of anxiety. Trigger points can also be activated by lifting heavy weights overhead, push-ups, severe coughing, or poor posture.

TECHNIQUES FOR WORKING THE SERRATUS ANTERIOR

This muscle should be worked in all positions, supine, side-lying, and prone. I find the side-lying position offers the most advantages for access. The serratus lies on top of the ribs, not in between. Most tender areas and trigger points are found on the upper ribs and the lateral ribs along the line of the nipple. Work the muscle from the ribs toward the shoulder blade, which promotes proper scapula placement and encourage your client to breathe into the lateral ribs to expand them while you work.

The photos show the side-lying position. To access the serratus in the supine and prone positions, slide in front of the anterior/lateral edge of latissimus dorsi. Press directly on the ribs. Follow the instructions for side-lying position.

In the Side-Lying Position:

1. **Skin Rolling:** Start by skin rolling without lubricant which helps to release the connective tissue (fascia).Have the client position her arm out of your way by propping on a small pillow.

2. **Latitudinal stroking:** Anterior to posterior along the ribs, to encourage length in this often locked short muscle.

3. **Pin and Move:** Locate tender spots and trigger points and release with static compression and deep stroking. **Active protraction and retraction** of the scapula by reaching the arm across the body and back is quite effective for releasing this stubborn muscle.

In the *photo right* the therapist is working over the client's sports bra, but it's easy to drape the client to just expose the ribs.

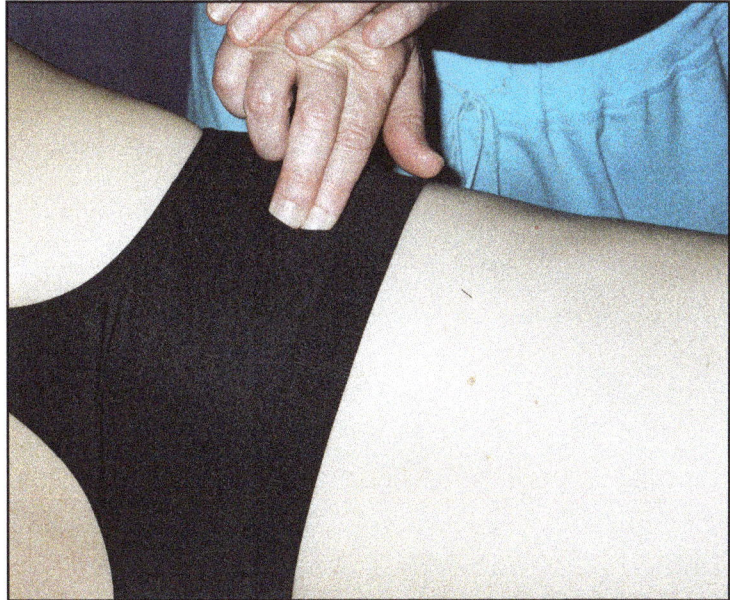

Locating tender spots and trigger points in the side-lying position.

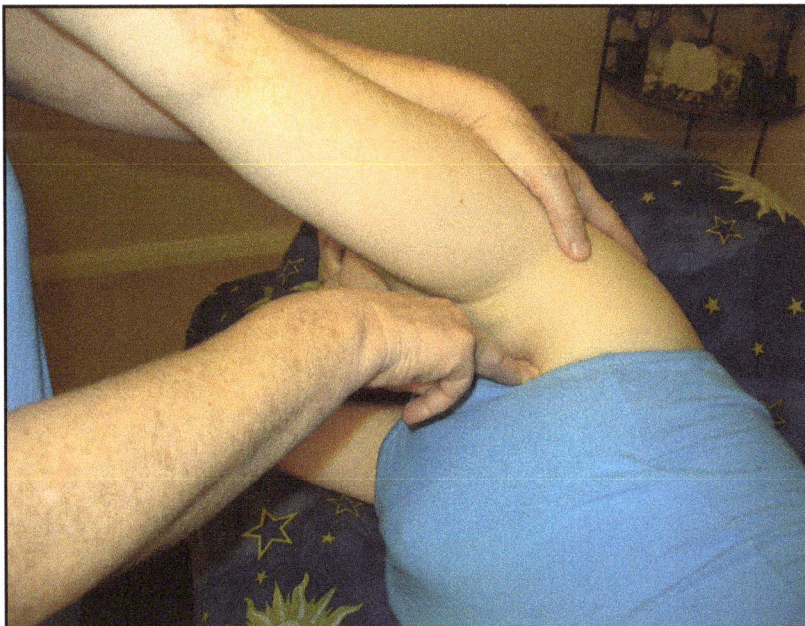

Releasing the superior fibers of the serratus in the side-lying position.

4. **Releasing the Superior Fibers:** To release the superior fibers of the serratus, place your fingers as if you were accessing subscapularis. Instead of pressing towards the scapula, press your fingers on the upper ribs.

Again, have your client reach her arm across her body and back as you release trigger points and hot spots.

5. SERRATUS ANTERIOR STRETCH:

Client is side-lying on the side opposite of the one to be stretched. Press the shoulder blade into full retraction (adduction). This is a subtle stretch but clients with a tight serratus will find it quite pleasant.

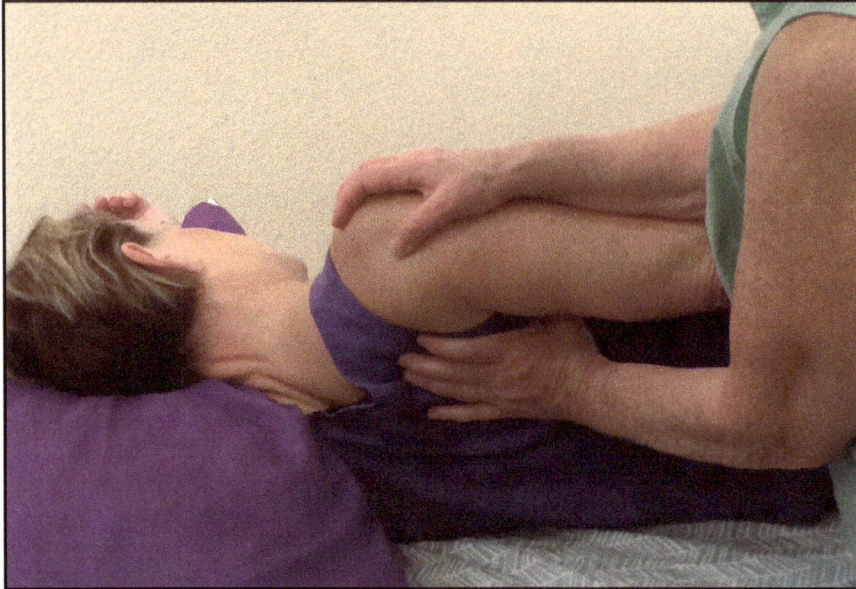

Serratus Stretch:
side view

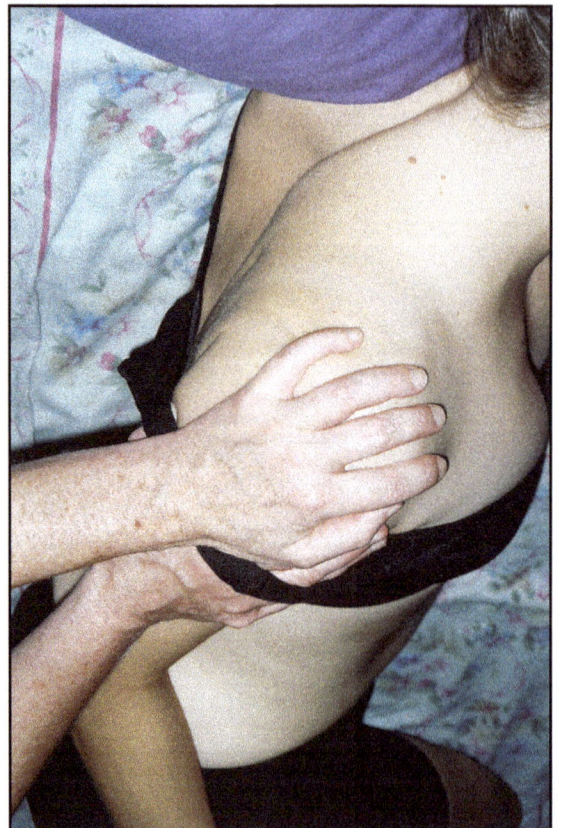

Serratus Stretch:
view from above

Practice patience, non-judgment, curiosity, and compassion.

TRAPEZIUS MUSCLE

Actions: (upper fibers) elevation and upward rotation of the scapula; lateral flexion of the neck; extreme contralateral rotation of the neck; (middle fibers) retraction and upward rotation of the scapula; (lower fibers) depression and upward rotation of the scapula
Attachments: (upper fibers) : superior - occiput; inferior- nuchal ligament of cervical spine; lateral - outer third of the clavicle; (middle fibers): medially - spinous processes of C6 to T4; laterally - acromion and superior lip of the spine of the scapula; (lower fibers) : medially - spinous processes of T5 to T12; laterally - root of the spine of the scapula.

Since the trapezius upwardly rotates the scapula, tight traps can limit abduction of the humerus above 60-90 degrees. And who doesn't have tight traps?! These muscles are often the overlooked component in restoring full range of movement to the shoulder joint. Typically the upper traps are more developed than the lower traps, which means that the lower traps (which depress the scapula) cannot balance the upward pull of the upper traps on the scapula and clavicle. The middle traps are often weak and overstretched due to a slumped shoulder posture. Both the middle and lower traps usually benefit from strengthening exercises, which help stabilize the shoulder girdle and therefore release the load on the rotator cuff.

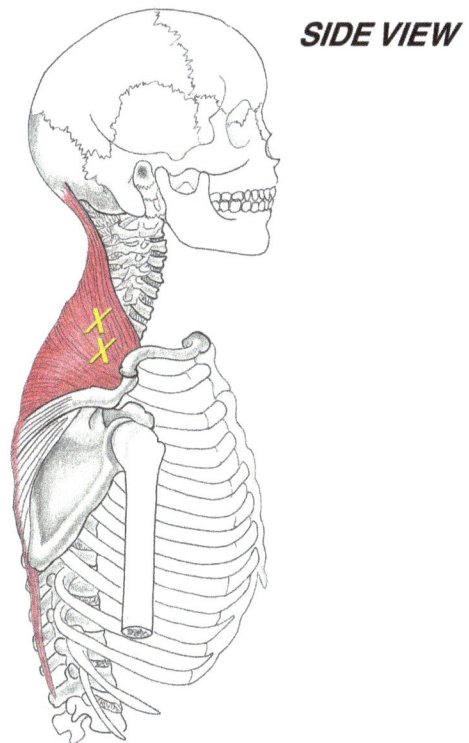

SIDE VIEW

The upper trapezius often gets enmeshed with the posterior scalene, which it sits on top of, in a dysfunctional relationship which inhibits healthy functioning of either muscle.

Trigger points refer to the shoulder, neck, side of the head, and sometimes down the arm, and are the most frequently activated trigger points in the body. Activation of trigger points is varied. The most common is the minimal antigravity function of the traps is overstressed by being forced to help carry the weight of the arm for long periods of time (holding the scapulae in an elevated position), and poor posture.

TECHNIQUES FOR WORKING THE ACROMIAL/CLAVICULAR ATTACHMENTS OF THE TRAPEZIUS

Since most massage therapists are quite capable in releasing the trapezius, the following protocol focuses on working the acromial/clavicular attachments. Work the entire muscle but concentrate on this usually overlooked area of glued tissue. Client can be supine, side-lying, or prone, but I find the supine position offers the best access. Concentrate your work in the small area around the attachments at the acromion process and the clavicle.

1. **Skin roll** the area to free up this often glued down tissue.

2. **Free the Attachments:** Perform deep parallel stripping, cross-fiber friction, and static pressure to free the attachments.

3. **Pin and Move:** If the client is able, have her **actively abduct** the humerus above 90 degrees while you work to engage the upward rotation action of trapezius. Make sure the shoulder joint is externally rotated during abduction.

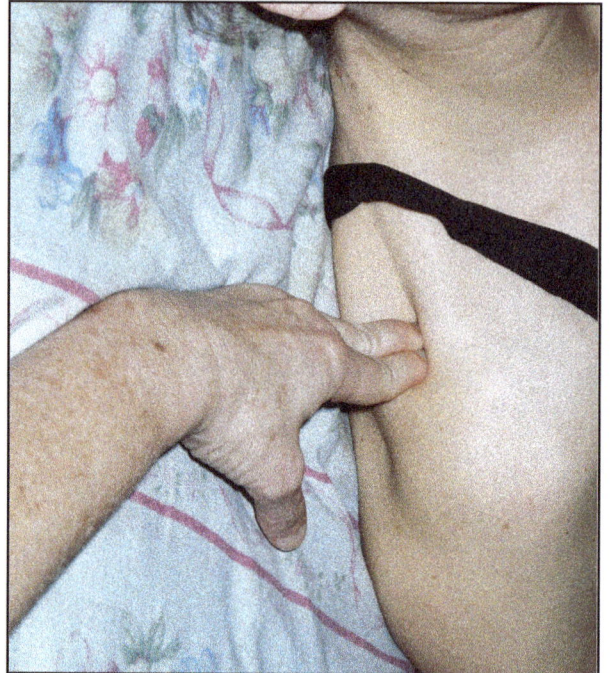

Overhead view of working the lateral attachments

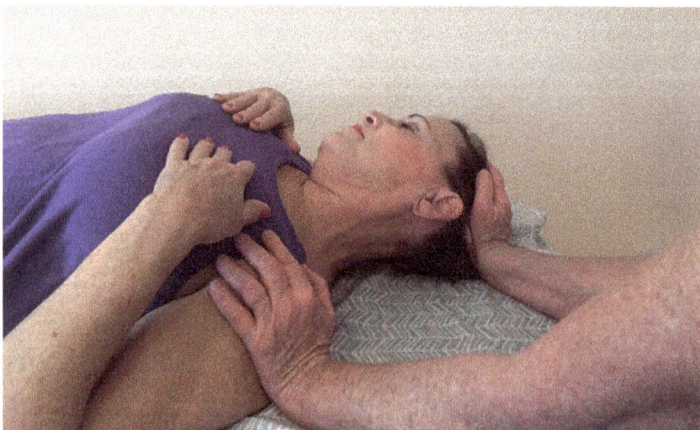

4. UPPER TRAPEZIUS STRETCH:

Client is supine. Therapist laterally flexes the neck (ear to shoulder). Ask the client to rotate her head *away* from the side of the neck being stretched. The degree of rotation is important - the neck should be rotated at least 50 degrees. In the *photo left*, the therapist's right hand is gently pushing the client's right shoulder down while the left hand is gently pressing the head and neck towards the left shoulder.

Latissimus Dorsi And Teres Major Muscles

Actions: internally rotates, extends, and adducts the humerus at the shoulder joint.
Attachments: Latissimus: inferior - thoracolumbar aponeurosis, lower three or four ribs, inferior angle of the scapula; superior - bicipital groove of the humerus.
Teres Major: inferior - inferior angle and lateral border of the scapula; superior -bicipital groove of the humerus (joins with the latissimus).

The latissimus dorsi and teres major are two other internal rotators of the shoulder joint that tend to be locked short and require release and stretching. Restriction in either of these muscles pulls the scapula downward, inhibiting the mobility of the shoulder girdle and the ability of the humerus to reach up and forward.

Trigger points refer to the mid-back around the inferior angle of the scapula, the posterior deltoid, and the side of the abdomen. Trigger points can be activated by lifting heavy weights, repetitive reaching forward and upward, and poor posture.

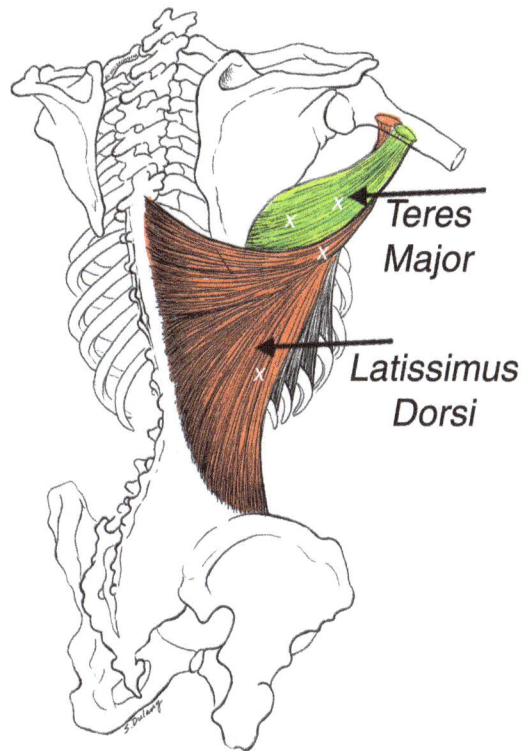

Teres Major

Latissimus Dorsi

Techniques For Working The Latissimus Dorsi And Teres Major

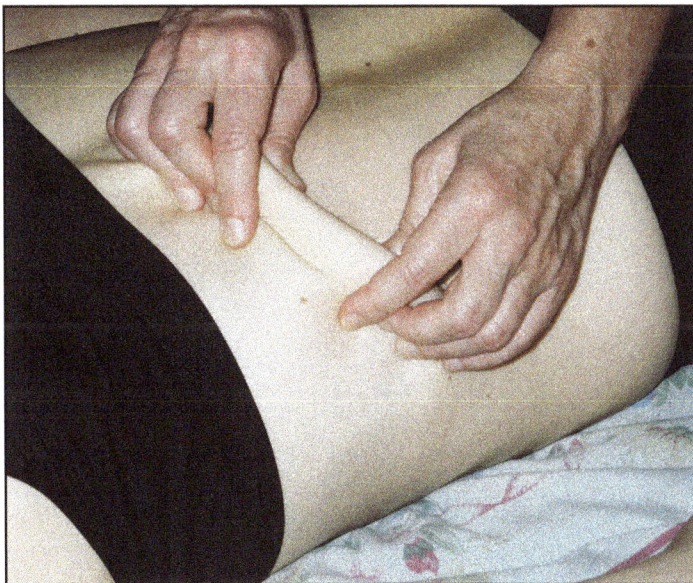

1. **Skin Rolling:** Client is prone. Skin rolling helps to release the connective tissue (fascia). If you've already applied lubricant, simply wipe off with a towel. As you skin roll, feel for places where the skin won't give. Those are areas where the connective tissue is "glued" down. These areas will feel tender to your client. Gently work to unglue the areas.

57

2. **Muscle Stripping:** Perform lengthening strokes, releasing the latissimus at the sacral and iliac crests. This will help to release the scapula from the downward pull of the latissimus. Work in line with the direction of the muscle fibers.

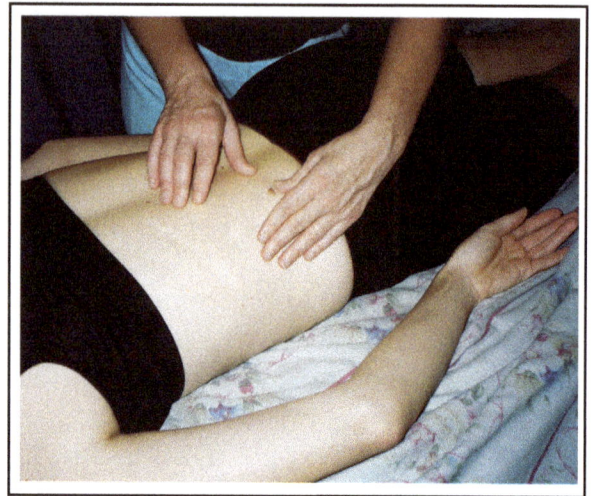

3. **Pinch the wad of muscle** behind the armpit with the fingers and thumb and release the attachment of these muscles where they join together on the humerus. *The photo left shows this in the supine position. You can also do it in the prone position. I usually do this after working the subscapularis in the supine position.*

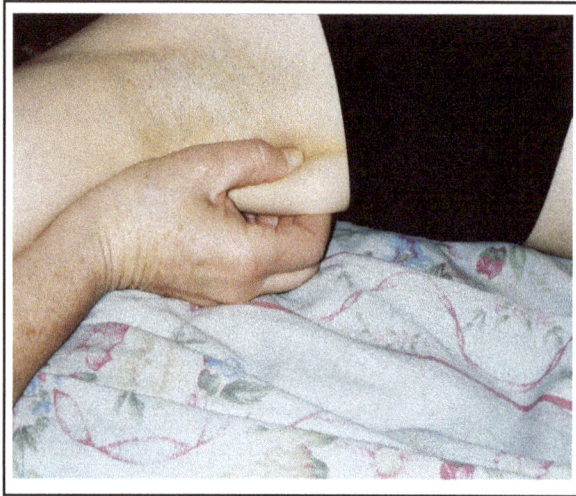

4. LATISSIMUS/TERES MAJOR STRETCH:

Client is side-lying on the side *opposite* of the one to be stretched. The therapist abducts the arm to just behind the head. If the client finds it painful to bring the arm behind the head, which requires a large degree of external rotation of the humerus, allow the arm to rest where it's comfortable. Press the arm down towards the table while gently pulling the arm away from the hip in a tractioning move. Use your other hand to stabilize the torso and press the illiac crest away from the ribs.

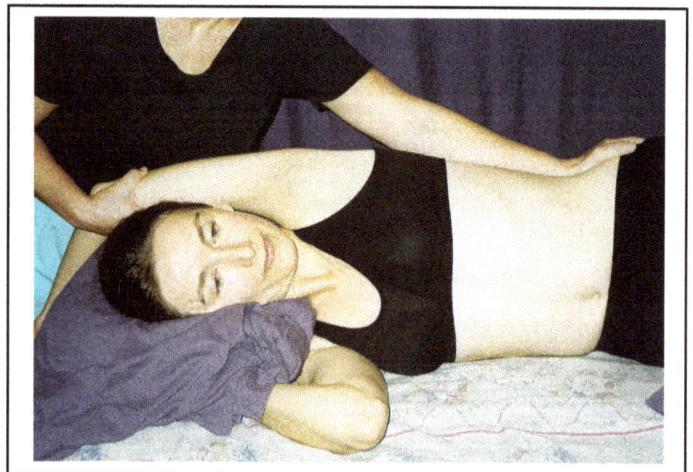

Client

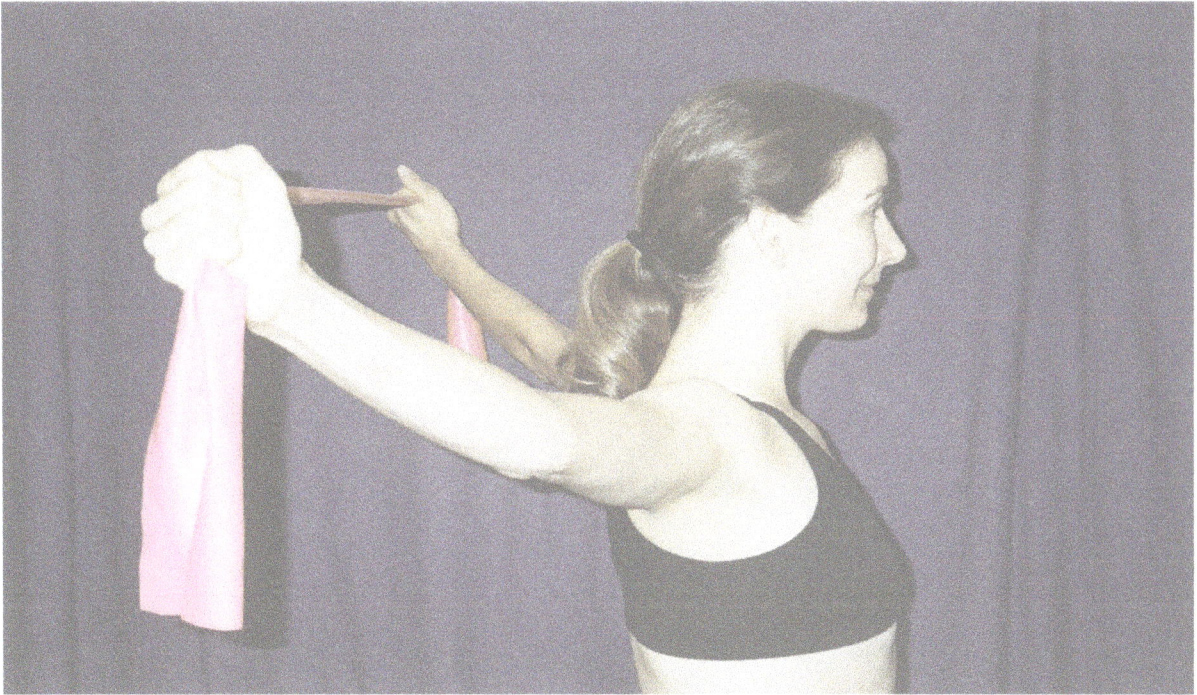

Education

CLIENT EDUCATION

An educated client will appreciate your for the rest of their life!

This section contains suggestions for sleep position and stretches your clients can do at home. Feel free to make copies of these pages as hand-outs for your clients.

For a more in-depth look at this subject written for the lay-person see my *From Ouch to Aaah!" Shoulder Pain Self-Care* book which allows your clients to "take you home" with them and extend the benefits of your healing touch. For more information go to the link below:

https://www.massagepublications.com/from-ouch-to-aaah/

SLEEP POSITIONING:

A client can re-injure or aggravate her shoulder by improper sleep positioning. It is essential to discuss this topic with your client and instruct her on how to position herself while sleeping. It can take several months to change and integrate a new position. Sleeping on the back is fine as long as she doesn't cross her arms over her face or allow the shoulders to rest on the pillow - the shoulders should rest on the bed. The goal is to keep the shoulder joint in **neutral** as much as possible during sleep.

Photos A and B below show correct and incorrect side-lying sleep positions.

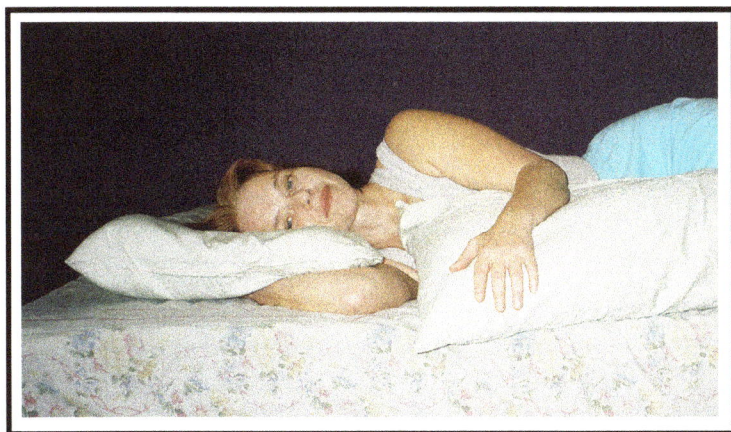

A. Correct use of a pillow to prevent shortening of the right subscapularis muscle (lower arm in L shape under the pillow) and stretching of the left infraspinatus and teres minor muscles (top arm resting in neutral on the pillow).

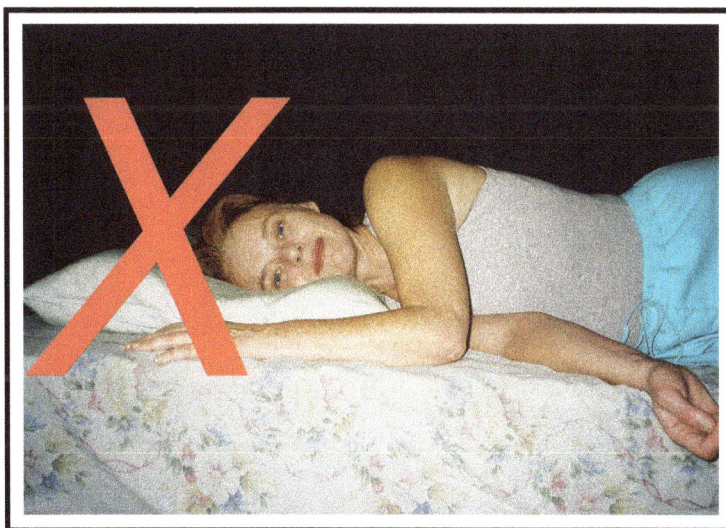

B. Incorrect use of a pillow. This position shortens the right subscapularis muscle (lower arm is held in an internally rotated position) and places the left (upper arm) infraspinatus and teres minor muscles in a pain producing stretch.

PENDULUM EXERCISE: An excellent, gentle, releasing exercise for the shoulder joint is to come into a lunge position and allow the affected arm to hang down toward the floor. Circle that arm (imagine drawing small circles on the floor with your fingers) clockwise then counterclockwise. Even better is to use a hand weight, anywhere from five to ten pounds. This tractions the head of the humerus which tends to get jammed up in the joint.

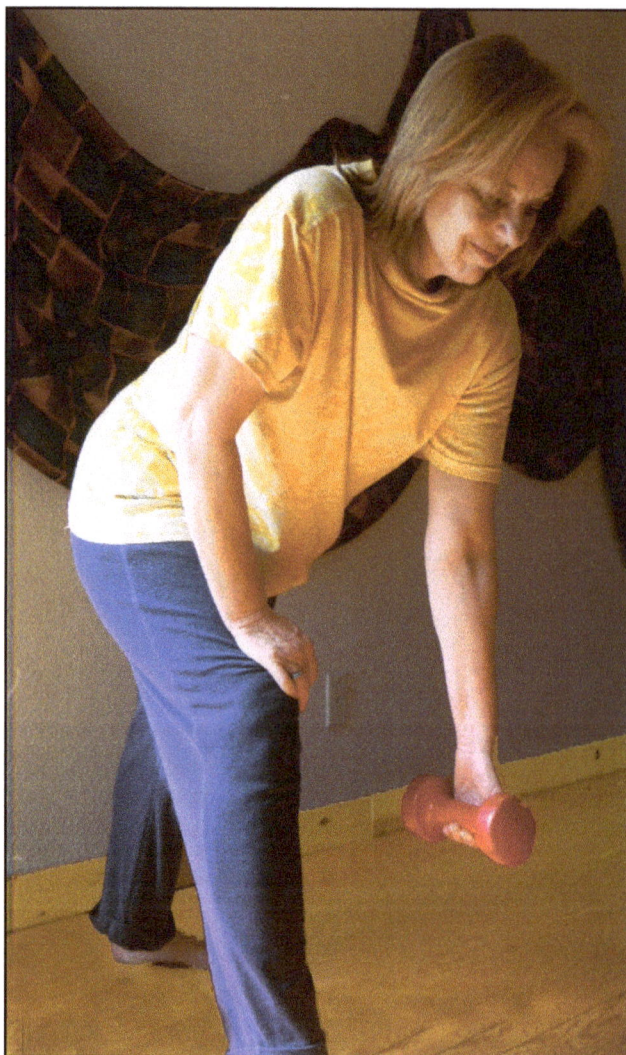

SELF-STRETCHES

THORACIC SPINE MOBILITY

Thoracic spine mobility is an extremely important, and often times overlooked, component to a variety of dysfunctions. Poor thoracic mobility can affect the shoulder, neck, low back, and hip very easily. Unfortunately, our daily habits and posture make us all very prone to poor thoracic spine mobility.

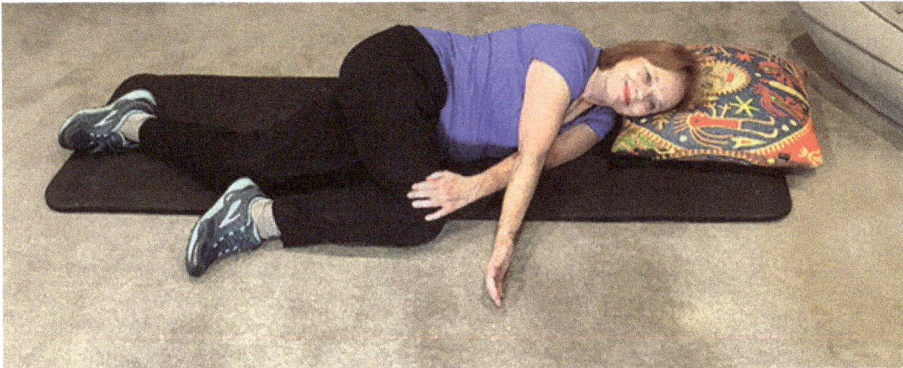

Step One:
- Lie on your side with your head supported by a pillow. Your bottom leg is straight. Your top leg is bent.
- Place the palm of your lower (the side you are lying on) hand on the knee of your top leg. Maintain that hand placement during the exercise.
- Place your top hand pinky down on the floor

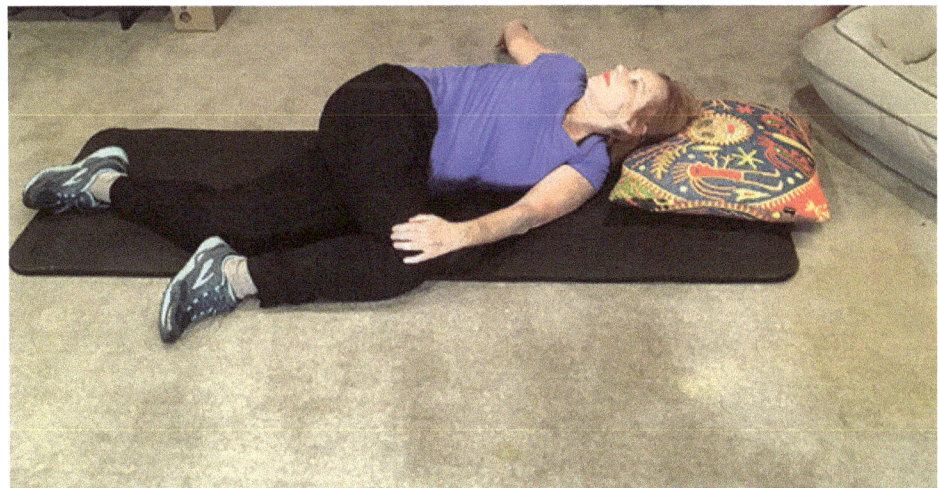

Step Two:
- Reach your top arm behind you, shoulder height and keep your palm up
- Allow your eyes to follow your hand.
- If your arm does not contact the floor, no problem! Don't force it - it will come in time. Do 5-10 reps each side.

Stretching the internal rotators is an absolute must for regaining a healthy balance between internal and external rotators of the shoulder joint and for good posture. Muscles that have been locked short will not allow a person to find an optimal posture and alignment of joints. Slow, gentle stretching re-educates these muscles. *All stretches should be held for at least 15 seconds or longer - 3-4 deep breaths.*

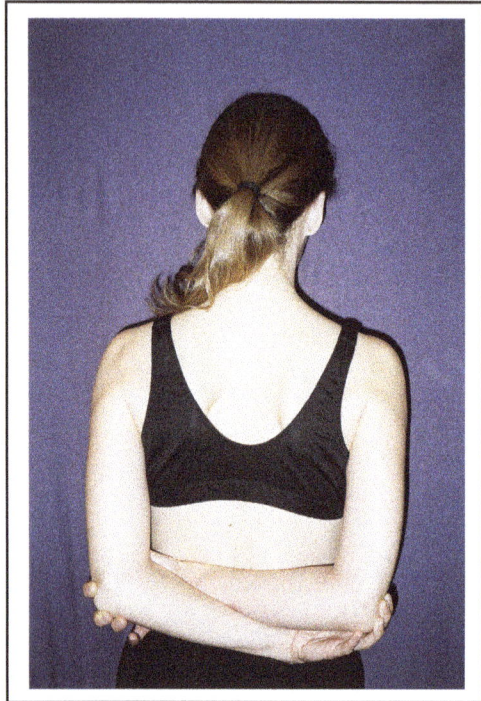

CRADLE THE ARMS BEHIND YOU STRETCH:
This is an excellent and gentle self-stretch for the pecs that can be done as many times during the day as possible, especially for someone who works at a computer. Cradle the arms behind by grasping the forearms or elbows, then squeeze the scapulae together.

*This stretch is only for those who can bring their arms behind the back with no pain.

OVER THE PILLOW STRETCH:
This is a wonderful self-stretch for the pecs and other internal rotators that can be done alone or assisted. Prop one or more pillows under the *mid-back* so the head is in hyperextension, yet supported by the table, bed, or floor. The number of pillows depends on the flexibility of your client (or yourself). For a client with limited flexibility, start with one pillow then build up. Make sure the shoulders are externally rotated. **The arms can be over the head or out to the side, depending on flexibility.** This stretch is also great for deepening the breath. The client

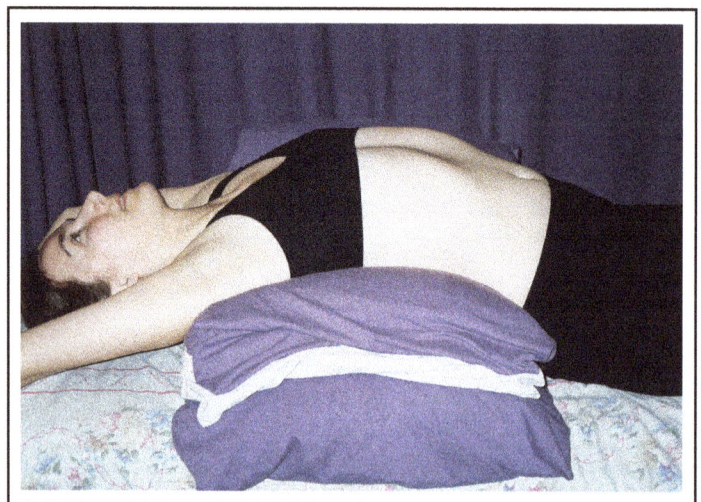

will also be getting a gentle sternocleidomastoid stretch. This has the added benefit of gently increasing hyperextension of the spine.

WALL STRETCH:

This is an easy stretch that can be done anywhere there is a wall!

■ Start by placing your bent elbow against a wall. The humerus is abducted to 90 degrees (shown) or higher. The degree of abduction will shift the emphasis on different fibers of the pec major and other internal rotators.

■ Leaving the elbow in place, turn your body, including your feet, away from your elbow. Hold for 15-25 seconds and repeat on the other side.

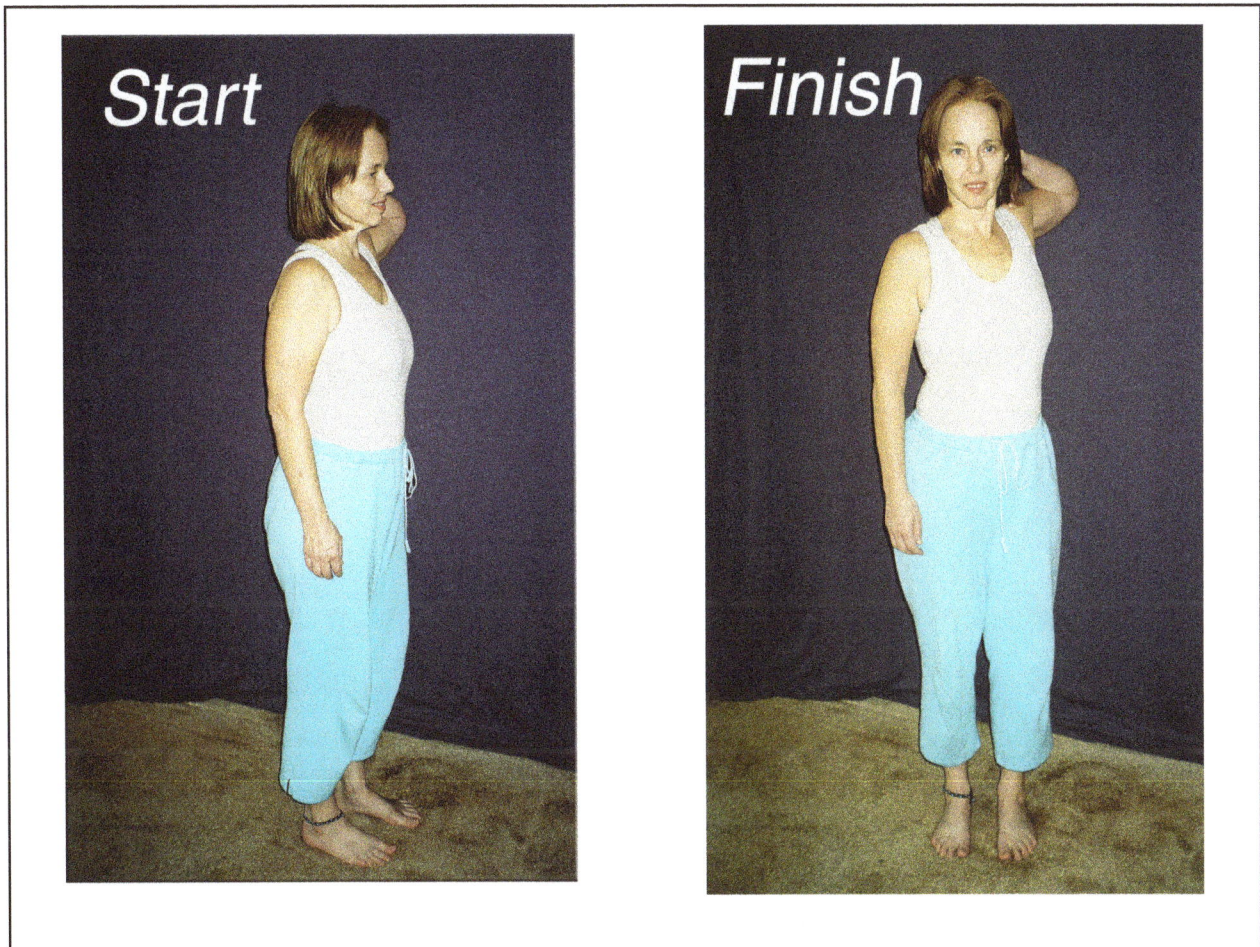

Errors to avoid:

■   Internally rotating the shoulder joint. Maintain external rotation.
■   Walking the feet away from the wall. Keep the body in a straight "column."

Band Stretch:

This stretch can be done with a thera-band, towel, scarf, or belt. The band allows the most versatility.

■   Place your hands on either end of the band, and lift your arms up over your head. Shrug your shoulders up, then let them fall down.

■   *Level One:* slowly press your arms back, keeping the elbows straight but not locked. Hold for 15-25 seconds. Repeat 3 to 5 repetitions.

■   *Level Two:* for a more intense stretch **(not recommended for the early stages of recovery)**, bring the arms down behind the back, then back up to starting position. Hold for 15-25 seconds. Repeat 3 to 5 repetitions.

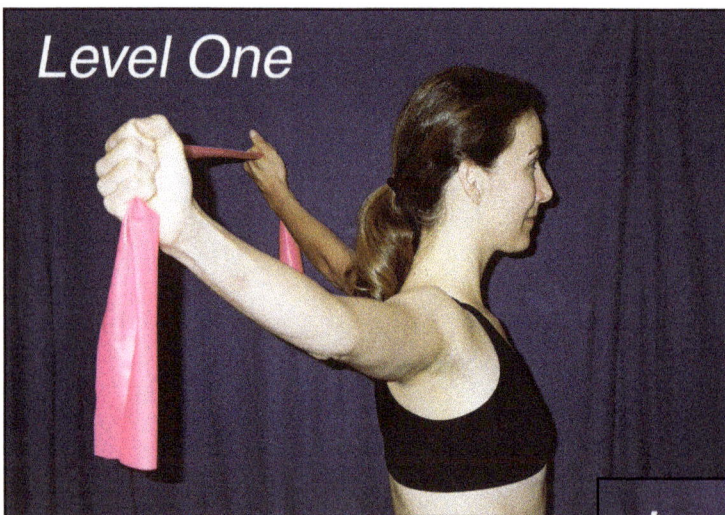

Level One

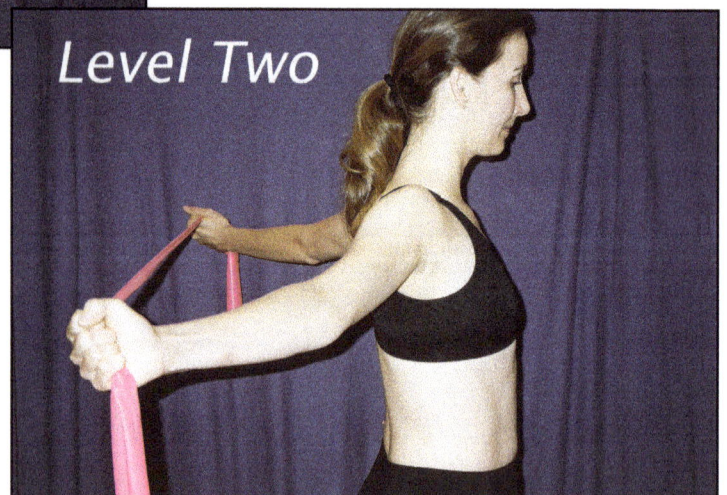

Level Two

Errors to avoid:

■   Internally rotating the shoulder joint. Maintain external rotation.
■   Allowing the pelvis to tip forward. Maintain neutral lumbar alignment.

BROOMSTICK STRETCH:

This is a great stretch that targets the subscapularis. The photos below show the left subscapularis being stretched.

■To stretch the left subscapularis, place a broomstick behind the back, grasp the pole end with the left hand, palm facing out with the humerus abducted 90 degrees.

■The right hand gently pushes the broom end forward which increases the degree of external rotation.

To stretch the right subscapularis, reverse the instructions. Maintain neutral alignment of the spine.

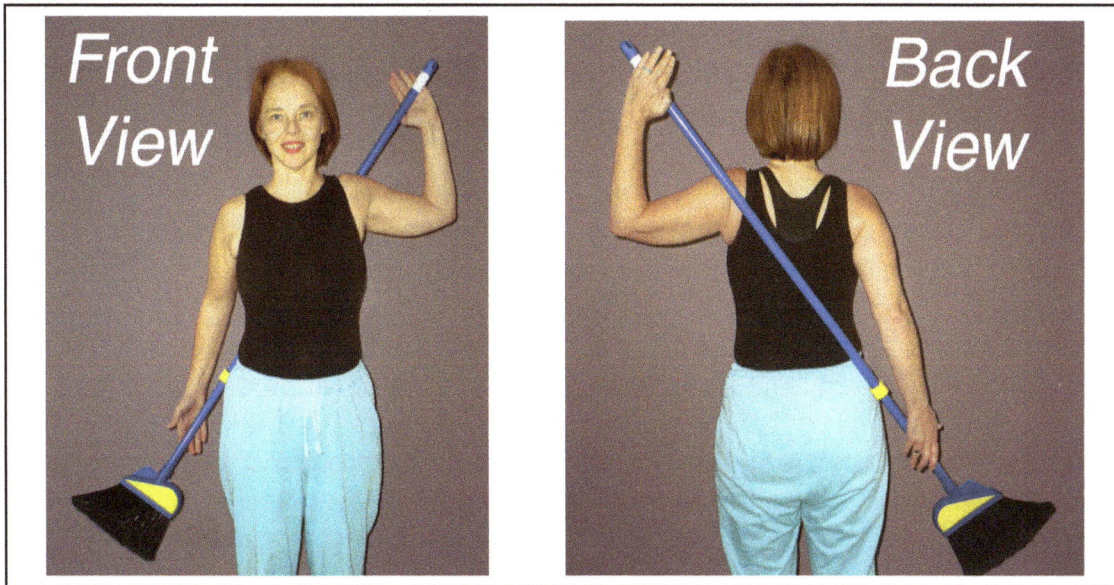

SUPRASPINATUS STRETCH:

The photo right shows the left supraspinatus being stretched.

Grasp the forearm of the side you want to stretch and slowly pull it across the back.

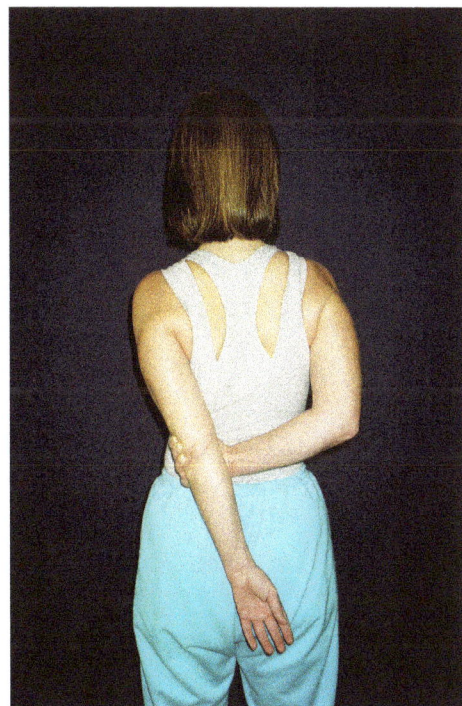

Errors to avoid:
- ■ Internally rotating the shoulder joint.
- ■ Maintain external rotation.

Additional Suggestions

1. Suggest that your client lie supine on the floor with the arms in a **"T"** position at least once a day. This encourages the opening of the chest and external rotation of the shoulder joint with the body being supported by the floor and not weight bearing. To intensify this, a bolster can be placed either vertically along the spine, or horizontally across the spine at the level of the lower edge of the scapulae. If necessary, bend knees and place feet flat on the floor.

2. Have your client slip her thumbs through her belt loops on the sides of her hips, which places the shoulders in a neutral position.

3. Swimming the back stroke is an excellent rehabilitation exercise for rotator cuffs. Even if your client doesn't like to swim, encourage her to do the backstroke in a standing position. You can even do it with your client after the session.

4. If your client has restricted range of motion, holding a six-inch ball between the elbow and side for several minutes can help. Have the client focus on pushing the ribs out into the ball with each inhalation as she presses the ball into her arm and tractions the forearm by gently pulling it with the opposite hand. She then can move the ball all the way up into the armpit, visualizing separating the clavicle, scapula, and humerus. This can create space in the shoulder joint and help release some of tightness in the surrounding soft tissue.

5. When carrying heavy objects, keep the elbows close to the side.

6. Always raise the arm away from the side (abduction) with the thumb up.

> For a more in-depth look at this subject written for the lay-person see my *From Ouch to Aaah!" Shoulder Pain Self-Care* book which allows your clients to "take you home" with them and extend the benefits of your healing touch. For more information go to the link below:

https://www.massagepublications.com/from-ouch-to-aaah/

Visualizations For Happy Movement

If we look at rotator cuff injuries globally, we'll find that incorrect body mechanics and movement contribute to this condition. Good posture and movement are essential to a vibrant, healthy, and enjoyable life. To consistently ignore our body requires enormous repressive energies. To learn more about our body, to use it more efficiently and for more activities, requires constant attention to the creation of new movements and the novel sensations they bring.

Movement allows us to feel alive, vital, and passionate about life. When we move in a variety of ways, different parts of our nervous system are stimulated, giving us a new sense of ourselves, a fresh identity. Below are some visualizations that I've collected over the years from many sources to encourage a new and happy sense of movement.

◆   *Imagine you have a feather attached vertically at the back of your head. As you move your head let the feather draw shapes in the sky.*

◆   *Visualize your neck as an incredibly long, golden, flexible coil of taffy that can move effortlessly in many directions. Discover where your coil can go and cannot go. Feel the pliability and agility as they increase in your neck.*

◆   *Imagine the skull as a big vertebra sitting on top of the spine.*

◆   *Imagine that your arms are beautiful white wings. As you move them, feel the wind lifting and lowering your arms.*

◆   *As you inhale deeply, feel your ribs expanding to the sides of the room, gently touching the walls. At the same time, experience and visualize the lengthening of your spine as if it were an elegant redwood tree extending high into the sky.*

◆   *Visualize your breath as having a color. See that color of breath filling up your entire chest, horizontally and vertically as you inhale. Sense your clavicles being gently widened by the breath color inside you.*

◆   *As you inhale and exhale, visualize your ribs moving like an accordion as your lungs expand and contract. The accordion closes on the exhale and opens on the inhale. Enjoy the stretch from inside.*

◆   *Create more range of motion at the sternoclavicular joint by imagining the clavicles opening and widening out into space.*

◆   *Imagine a flower in the center of your chest. As you inhale, let the flower open up farther and farther until you can smell the fragrance.*

HAPPY EXPLORATIONS!

——————————————●——————————————

References And Suggested Reading

Austin, Derek R. PT DPT MS BCTMB CSCS; Haun, Jolie, PhD EdS LMT; Gillespie Pualani, LMT MS RN BCTMB. Massage Reduces Non-Specific Shoulder Pain and Improves Function. Massage Today. April 2015. Volume 15

Beach, Zakary M, Tucker, Jennica J, Thomas, Stephen J., Reuther, Katherine E., Gray, Chancellor F, Chang-Soo Lee, David L. Glaser, Louis J. Soslowsky. Biceps tenotomy in the presence of a supraspinatus tear alters the adjacent intact tendons and glenoid cartilage. Journal of Biomechanics. 2017

Bennell, Kim, Wee, Ellen, Coburn, Sally, Green, Sally, Harris, Anthony, Staples, Margaret, Forbes, Andrew, Buchbinder, Rachelle: Efficacy of Standardized Manual Therapy and Home Exercise Program for Chronic Rotator Cuff Disease: Randomized Placebo Controlled Trial; BMJ 2010; 340:c2756 doi:10.1136/bmj.c2756

Benjamin, Ben, Ph.d; The Forgotten Rotator Cuff, Part 1; Massage Today; February, 2014, Vol. 14, Issue 02.

Benjamin, Ben, Ph.d; The Forgotten Rotator Cuff, Part 2; Massage Today; April, 2014, Vol. 14, Issue 04.

Burkhart, Steven S, MD & Tehrany, Armin M, MD: Arthroscopic Subscapularis Tendon Repair: Technique and Preliminary Results, Arthroscopy: The Journal of Arthroscopic and Related Surgery; Volume 18 #5 2002

Chaitow, Leon, ND, DO. Positional Release Techniques: What are the Mechanisms? Massage Today. January 2016, Volume 16, Issue 01

Conable, Barbara: How to Learn the Alexander Technique, Andover Press, 1991,

Davies, Clair: The Trigger Point Therapy Workbook, New Harbinger Publications, Inc., 2001.

Davies, Clair: The Frozen Shoulder Workbook: Trigger Point Therapy for Overcoming Pain and Regaining Range of Motion; New Harbinger Publications; 2006.

Dalton, Erik: Finding the Weak Key Link – Kinetic Chain Assessment. Massage and Bodywork, March/April 2014

Earls, James, Myers, Thomas: Fascial Release for Structural Balance; North Atlantic Books; 2010.

Gibbons, John. (2016) Muscle energy techniques: A practical guide for physical therapists. Chichester, Eng.: Lotus Pub.

Hamill, Joseph & Knutzen, Kathleen: Biomechanical Basis of Human Movement, Lippincott, Williams & Williams, 1995

Hidalgo-Lozano, Amparo; Fernández-de-las-Peñas, César; Díaz-Rodríguez, Lourdes; González-Iglesias, Javier, et al.: Changes in pain and pressure pain sensitivity after manual treatment of active trigger points in patients with unilateral shoulder impingement: A case series. Journal of Bodywork and Movement Therapies Vol. 15, Issue 4, Pages 399-404 October 2011

Horrigan, Joseph & Robinson, Jerry: The 7-Minute Rotator Cuff Solution, Health for Life, 1991.

Hwang,Kyu Rim, Murrell,George A.C., MD, DPhil, Millar, Neal L. PhD, FRCSEd

(Tr&Ortho), Bonar,Fiona, MBBCh, FRCPath, Lam, Patrick, PhD, Walton,Judie R. PhD. Advanced glycation end products in idiopathic frozen shoulders. Journal of Elbow and Shoulder Surgery. January 5, 2016.

Jae-Man Kwak, MDa, Tae-Hyun Ha, MSa, Yucheng Sun, MDb, Erica Kholinne, MDc, Kyoung-Hwan Koh, MD, PhDa, In-Ho Jeon, MD, PhDa. (2019). Motion quality in rotator cuff tear using an inertial measurement unit: new parameters for dynamic motion assessment. Journal of Shoulder and Elbow Surgery.

Kopf, Karl: Healthy Shoulder Handbook: 100 Exercises for Treating and Preventing Frozen Shoulder, Rotator Cuff and other Common Injuries; Ulysses Press; 2010.

Liebenson, Craig: The Serratus Punch. Journal of Bodywork and Movement Therapies Vol. 16, Issue 2, Pages 268-269. April 2012

Lowe, Whitney: Functional Assessment in Massage Therapy, 2nd edition, Pacific Orthopedic Massage, 1995.

Mandalidis , Dimitris; O'Brien Moira; :Relationship between hand-grip isometric strength and isokinetic moment data of the shoulder stabilisers.Journal of Bodywork and Movement Therapies Vol. 14, Issue 1, Pages 19-26. January 2010

Mörl ,Falk; Matkey , Andreas; Bretschneider , Susanne; Bernsdorf , Annette, et al.: Shoulder functionality after manual therapy in subjects with shoulder impingement syndrome: A case series. Journal of Bodywork and Movement Therapies Vol. 17, Issue 2, Pages 212-218. April 2013

Muscolino, Joseph, DC. Science and Technique: Deliver More Effective Bodywork. Massage and Bodywork Quarterly. March/April 2016.

Myers, Thomas: Anatomy Trains; Elsevier; 2008.

Newton, Don: Clinical Pathology for the Professional Bodyworker, Simran Publications, 1998.

Osar, Evan. (2018) Corrective Exercise Solutions to Common Hip and Shoulder Dysfunction. Chichester, Eng.: Lotus Publishing.

Østerås , Håvard, Myhr, Gunnar; Haugeru, Lasse; Torstensen, Tom Arild: Clinical and MRI findings after high dosage medical exercise therapy in patients with long lasting subacromial pain syndrome: A case series on six patients. Journal of Bodywork and Movement Therapies Vol. 14, Issue 4, Pages 352-360. October 2010

Porterfield, James A. & DeRosa, Carl: Mechanical Shoulder Disorders, Saunders Publishing, 2004.

Roberts, Debbie. Following a Road Less Traveled: Finding the cause of chronic shoulder pain where you least expect it. February, 2013, Vol. 13, Issue 02

Roberts, Debbie: Timing is Everything: Shoulder Instability and Labral Tears. Massage Today; December, 2013, Vol. 13, Issue 12

Roberts, Debbie: The Sub-Scap Attack. Massage Today; October, 2015, Vol. 15, Issue 10

Saithna, Adnan,BMedSci(Hons), MBChB, DipSEM, MSc, FRCS(T&O), Longo,Alison MS, Leiter, Jeff, PhD, Old, Jason MD, FRCSC, MacDonald, Peter M, MD, FRCS. Shoulder Arthroscopy Does Not Adequately Visualize Pathology of the Long Head of Biceps Tendon. Orthopaedic Journal of Sports Medicine January 2016 vol. 4 no. 1.

Schultz, R. Louis & Feitis, Rosemary: The Endless Web, North Atlantic Books, 1996,

Smith, Mary Atkinson, FNP & Smith, W. Todd, MD: Rotator Cuff Tears: An Overview, Orthopaedic Nursing • September/October 2010 • Volume 29 • Number 5

Totora, Gerald (2012) Principles of Human Anatomy and Physiology, 13th editioin. John Wiuley and Sons, Hoboken, NJ

Travell, Janet & Simons, David: Myofascial Pain and Dysfunction - The Trigger Point Manual, Volumes 1 & 2, William & Wilkins, 1983 (vol. 1), 1992 (vol. 2)).

Trundle, Terry, PTA, ATC, LAT,: Rotator Cuff Syndrome: From Impingement to Post Operative Rehab, Cross Country Education; 2009

Weber, Stephen MD; Chahal, Jaskarndip MD, MSc, MBA. (2019) Management of Rotator Cuff Injuries. Journal of the American Academy of Orthopaedic Surgeons

Zake, Yamuna & Golden, Stephanie: Body Rolling. Healing Arts Press, 1997.

Index

ABOUT THE AUTHOR

Peggy Lamb will tell you she is a massage therapist. She is a massage therapist, but she is so much more than that. When Peggy confronts a problem, she doesn't just solve the problem for herself. She will solve the problem for others, and try to insure that the problem isn't a problem for all her clients. When she tore a rotator cuff, she learned about shoulders, about how they move, how the function, and how they function well. Not only did she completely recover from her injury, she wrote a book "Releasing the Rotator Cuff" so other massage therapists can help their clients with shoulder injuries. When faced with a back injury, Peggy worked to recover from that, and recover she did. Not content to just overcome her own injury, she wrote another book "The Core of the Matter", with content geared to help others, and other massage therapists, with back problems. Peggy doesn't just fix issues that come up in her life, but she fixes those issues for others. Peggy Lamb is not just a massage therapist, she is an author of five books, a creator of four instructional DVDs , a teacher of massage therapists, a leader in her field. All of this comes from one feeling….. the desire to touch, to heal, and to be touched.

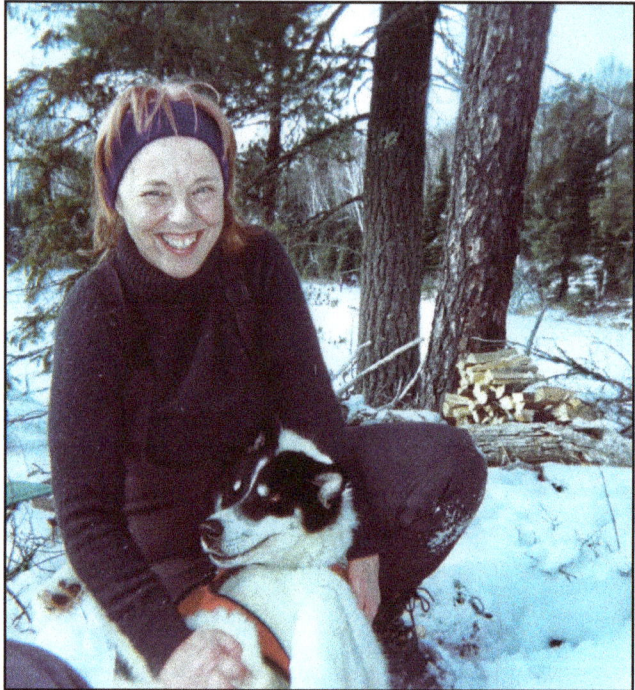

Peggy has practiced massage since 1986 and is nationally certified. She currently owns a private massage and movement therapy business, where she practices when she's not teaching. Peggy received her initial training at the New Mexico Academy of Massage and Advanced Healing Arts in Santa Fe, New Mexico, and at Wellness Skills, Inc., in Dallas, Texas. She taught clinical anatomy and physiology, Trigger Point therapy and Swedish technique at Wellness Skills, Inc., in Dallas and at Texas Healing Arts Institute in Austin.

In addition to her extensive training in massage therapy, Peggy holds a master's degree in Dance from American University in Washington, D.C. She has volunteered for 10 years with Truth be Told, teaching creative movement and writing to incarcerated women. Peggy brings her eclectic and extensive background into her teaching for an interesting, enjoyable and enlightening learning experience. When she's not working, Peggy can be found dancing, swimming in Austin's Barton Springs, hiking or even dog sledding.

Peggy is an approved CE provider for the Texas Department of Health, the National Certification Board for Therapeutic Massage and Bodywork, and the Florida Department of Health.